WORK THE PROBLEM

How I Became the Ringmaster of My Three-Ring
Circus

ROBERT CUMMER

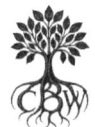

WORK THE PROBLEM

How I Became the Ringmaster of My Three-Ring Circus

by Robert Cummer

ISBN: 979-8-9934979-9-0 (Paperback)

ISBN: 979-8-9934979-8-3 (EPUB)

Published by:

Mangrove Publishing LLC

Midland, MI 48642

United States of America

Printed in the United States of America

For my Family and Friends
Thank you

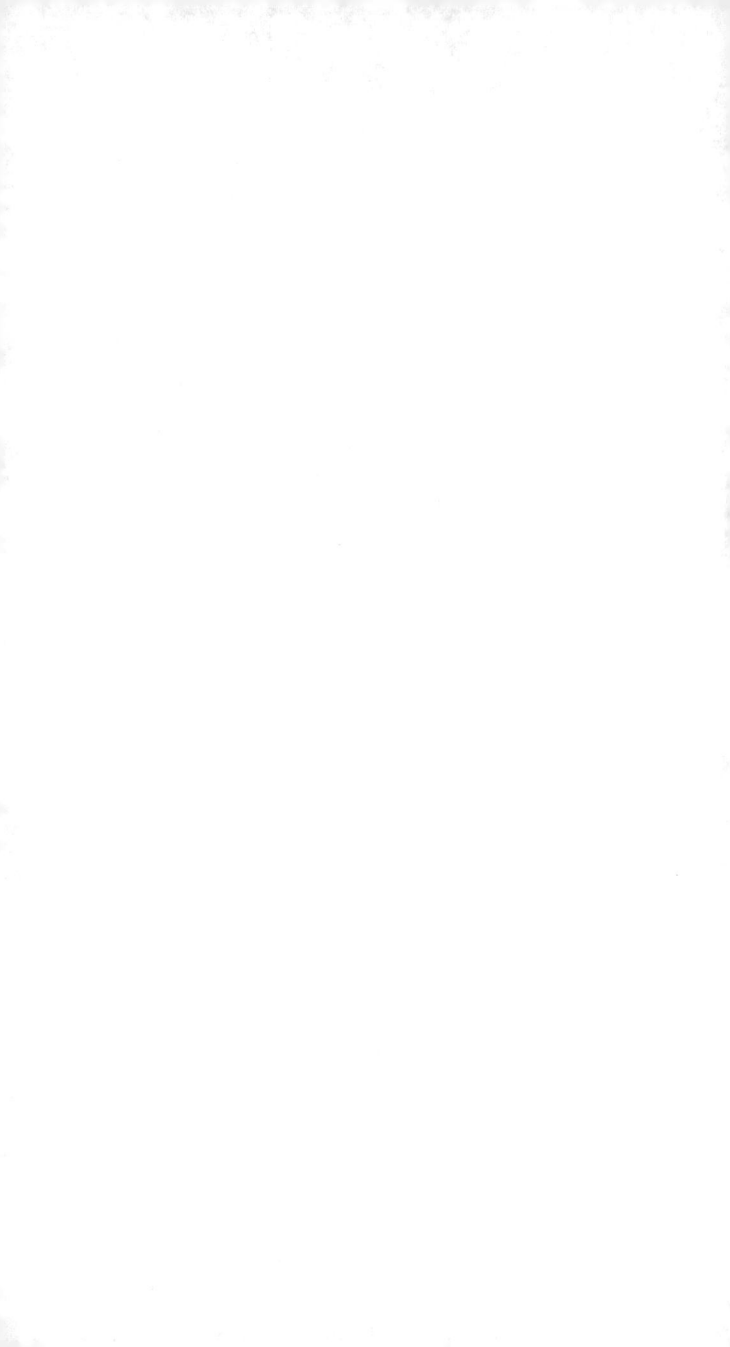

Preface

If open-heart surgery is anywhere on your timeline—before or after—this is written for you. And if you're here because you're just curious about what happened to me, I guess that's fine too.

Let's get a few things straight: This isn't medical advice. I'm not a doctor. I'm not selling a program. I'm not here to tell you to eat kale, forgive the universe, and wake up at 4:00 a.m. to "win the day." If that's your thing, great. This isn't that book.

Professionally, I've done everything from sorting returnable bottles (you won't find that on my recent resume) and stocking shelves at a grocery store, to working as an engineering technician, an automation engineer, and an entrepreneur. I have solved problems for a living my whole life. When something breaks, I work the problem: isolate variables, test assumptions, verify what's true, and try not to lie to myself about the data.

That's the lens I brought into heart disease, cardiac catheterizations, and eventually open-heart surgery.

I'm writing this because I didn't understand how surreal this experience is until I was in it. In fact, I'm not sure I even truly understood what the word *surreal* meant. The dictionary says "bizarre" or "dream-like," but those are just words. There's a difference between knowing something is serious and feeling its seriousness. You can read the pamphlets, nod through appointments with your cardiologist, and tell people you're fine. Then one day you're in a gown and non-slip socks, someone's rolling you down a hallway under fluorescent lights, and if you are anything like me, the part of your brain that thinks it's in control starts to realize it has an out-of-office message.

That moment changed me.

Over a span of a few years, I had two heart caths. The first one showed that I had two blockages, but no stents were inserted, partly due to the blockage location and severity; we would just keep an eye on them. Then I had a second heart cath, and that ended the debate. Not because I suddenly became wise, but because the data got loud enough that even I couldn't pretend it was "probably fine."

And here's something I want to say out loud, because I know I'm not the only one who does it.

Even though I've always considered myself to be data-driven, I still lie to myself. I rationalize. I bargain. I move the goalposts. I tell myself, "I'm still functioning. I'm still working. I'm still traveling. I haven't dropped dead. So maybe it's not that bad." That's what denial looks like when you think you're smart enough to build a convincing argument.

The truth is, I wasn't playing craps. I was playing Russian roulette, and I had been lucky.

If you're anything like me, you'll recognize that voice. The one that can explain away anything as long as it keeps your life comfortable and unchanged. The voice that says, "I'll deal with it later." As you'll soon see, *later* is a dangerous word.

This book is my attempt to put the truth on paper, both for you and for me. I want someone facing this to feel less alone. I want someone recovering to see that the weird parts of the process are actually normal. I want someone who's months or years out and still doesn't feel quite right to realize they're not broken—they're adapting to something that rearranged their life.

You'll read some dark humor in here. Not because any of this is funny, but because humor is a pressure-release valve. It doesn't erase the reality. It just makes it possible to breathe or cope while you're in it.

You'll also likely notice the engineer brain show up everywhere: systems, failure modes, checklists, data integrity, the way I describe fear like it's a problem I can troubleshoot. That's not me trying to sound clever. That's just how I think. I've also learned to compartmentalize my issues. Troubleshooting and compartmentalization have been the main tools in my toolbox. Those are the tools I reached for when my body became the thing that needed troubleshooting.

This book is not a tell-all. Like all families, we dealt with issues before surgery and during recovery. You also have to recognize that your situation isn't all about you; everyone in your family and circle of friends is affected. I had tremendous support from my people, and I'm forever grateful for that. I'm also not going to pretend this experience turned me into a saint or a fitness model. I've made improvements. I've lost weight. I've changed some habits. I've also got plenty of room to keep working physically and mentally. If you're looking for a perfect example to follow, you won't find it here.

What you will find is an honest account of what it felt like to face open-heart surgery and live through the aftermath. Not just the medical part—the mental part. The waiting. The fear. The boredom. The identity shift. The strange calm some days and the surprise anger and sadness on others. The moments you don't tell people about because you don't want to scare them, or because you don't have words for it yet.

How to use this book is simple. Read it straight through like a story, or use it like a field manual.

If surgery is coming up, start at the beginning. Pay attention to the mental game more than the mechanics. The mechanics will be handled by professionals. The mental game is yours.

If you're home recovering, skip ahead to the recovery chapters and look for anything that helps you get through the next day, not the next decade.

If you're months or years out and still feel off—tired, anxious, numb, irritable, unmotivated, or just different—start where you are. You're not late. You're not weak. You're not crazy. You're adapting.

I wrote this because I don't want to leave things on the table. Heart surgery has a way of clarifying what matters and what doesn't. It made me stop waiting for "someday." It made me start doing things I'd been carrying around for years without committing to. One of those things was writing. That doesn't mean my life became perfect. It means I got more honest about time.

If any part of this helps you—if it steadies you on a bad day, gives you language for what you're feeling, or makes you feel like you're sitting with somebody who gets it—then it did what I wrote it to do.

Let's get into it.

PART I
Before, During, After

This part is the event.

The before, the during, and the first stretch after—when everything is loud and nothing makes sense.

I'm writing it straight because that's the only way I know.

ONE

The One Percent

It is 3:00 AM on Thursday, January 19th, 2023.

My alarm is set for 3:30 AM, but I'm not asleep. How could I be? The house is quiet—the heavy winter silence you only get in Michigan in January. In two hours, I'm expected to be at St. Mary's Hospital on the east side of Saginaw, getting prepped for a double coronary artery bypass graft.

The doctors call it a CABG. The nurses call it "cabbage," like a grocery item they'll pick up on the way home. I call it the moment I lose control.

For the first time in my adult life, I'm about to hand over the keys to my existence to a room full of people I've just met. I'm a process control engineer by trade; my career has been built on understanding systems, managing variables, predicting outcomes. But lying here in the dark, I know the variables are no longer mine to manage.

The surgeon told me it's a "routine procedure." He sat in his office, calm and professional, and gave me the odds: approximately a 97% to 98% chance of success.

That sounds great to a layman. It sounds like an A-plus on a test.

But then he mentioned the inverse: approximately a 1% mortality rate.

Wait a minute, my brain fired back. One percent?

Most people hear 99% success and hear "guaranteed." I hear "statistical deviation." I know what a bell curve looks like. I know tails exist. And I know that if 100 people go into that operating room, one of them doesn't come home. The math doesn't care that I have a family. The math doesn't care that I have plans. The math just is.

I volunteered for this roller coaster ride.

Well—"volunteered" is a strong word. I was conscripted by biology and a cardiac cath image that looked like a roadmap to a dead end. But lying here, staring at the ceiling, I realize the ticket has already been punched.

This can't be real. There's no fucking way.

I keep saying it, but the words don't change anything. The clock still reads 3:05 AM. The surgery is still happening.

Twelve years earlier, I had an L4 to S1 back fusion. If something went wrong I could be paralyzed or I could talk more than I already do—it had risks. Something could go wrong. But at forty, I wasn't scared. I had waited ten years for that surgery—ten years of people looking at me like I was crazy when I described the pain. Two neurosurgeons. Multiple MRIs. Before one finally said, "Bob, we're going to do surgery."

When it was over, I asked him if I had been crazy. He said no. MRIs are static, he explained. They don't show movement. When he got in there, my vertebrae were loose—grinding. The pain was real.

But this is different.

This isn't my spine. This is the pump that feeds fresh oxygenated blood to everything. The thing that keeps everything else running. And in a few hours, they're going to stop it and let a machine take over that responsibility. Same with the lungs.

I run my hand over my chest. The skin is smooth. Intact.

This is the last time it will feel this way. I understood the procedure on paper. The surgeon explained it in his office. I knew what "open-heart" meant.

But knowing it and feeling it are different things. Lying there at 3:00 AM, it stopped being information and became reality. In a few hours they were going to saw through my sternum to get to my heart.

I also knew they'd harvest a vein from my leg. What I didn't understand—because nobody really can until it's yours—was what it would feel like afterward. The tenderness. The strange new limits. The healing that takes longer than you expect. And years later, the dead zones on my calves and chest where nerves were cut and never fully came back online.

I notice the sheets against my skin. Strange, the things you pay attention to when you're not sure you'll feel them again.

I wonder what my wife is really thinking. She's a trauma nurse. She knows exactly what's coming—the saw, the heart-lung machine, the hours of waiting while I'm on the table. Is she scared? She hasn't said it, but I know her well enough to know she's carrying more than she's showing.

I think about my kids. Are they lying awake somewhere too? Do they believe the 99%, or are they doing the same math I am?

My grandchildren are too young to understand. Most of them, anyway. They just know Papa isn't feeling well. They don't know Papa might not come home.

I wonder if my dogs would miss me.

Amusement park rides are generally safe. They have safety bars and inspections and track records. But every now and then, a bolt shears. A sensor fails.

I roll over and look at the clock. 3:07 AM.

The machine that is my body—the thoroughbred heart with the bad plumbing—is beating quietly in my chest. It doesn't know that in a few hours a saw is going to cut through the sternum to get to it. It doesn't know a team of strangers is going to stop it cold, hook me to a bypass machine, and run my blood through plastic tubing while they sew new routes around old blockages.

It was time to get my affairs in order. That phrase sounds so clinical. So tidy. But what does it actually mean?

It's not just paperwork. It's not just passwords and insurance policies.

It's the conversations. Did I say what needed to be said? Do my people know what they mean to me? Have I left any doubt?

I think about the home we made. I've always been proud of it. The life we built. The noise of grandchildren running through the rooms.

We didn't announce the surgery on social media. I wasn't looking for sympathy. That's not how I process things. Close friends and family knew, but I kept it tight. This was mine to carry.

The clock reads 3:12 AM. The countdown continues.

I don't know if you can ever be fully prepared for something like this. I'd read the material. I understood the mechanics as well as any engineer could without a medical degree. I trusted my surgeon. I'd passed all the tests— lungs, imaging, everything they needed before putting me under.

But lying here, I realize preparation only goes so far. There's a gap between knowing the facts and accepting what they mean.

All I know for certain is this: if I make it

through, I'm not leaving questions unanswered anymore. No more assuming people know how I feel. No more taking for granted there will be time later.

If I get another chance, I'm going to make sure the people I love never have to wonder.

The clock reads 3:15 AM.

I close my eyes. Not to sleep. Just to wait. But before I tell you what happened in that operating room, you need to know how I ended up on that calendar in the first place.

TWO

The Data Got Loud

For some bizarre reason, I'm a person that likes plenty of data—lots of data. I trust data. I also have a long, proud history of negotiating with data like it's a hostage situation. At one time early in my career, I was told by another engineer that was a true old-school statistician (paper and pencil calculations) that "figures lie and liars figure." That always stuck with me. I fell into both categories depending on what I was trying to rationalize. In this particular case, my cardio-vascular data.

For a while, my heart disease lived in that comfortable zone where you can pretend you're "managing" it. You can still work. Still travel. Still do normal things. You can tell yourself the story you want to hear: "They're watching it. It's hereditary. It's not cholesterol. It's fine." You can say "fine" with a straight face right up until the day the numbers stop letting you.

As I mentioned in the Preface, over a span of

a few years, I had two heart caths. The first one gave me something to watch. The second one was the moment the problem stopped being theoretical. It ended the debate, even though I still argued with it—because that's what I do. I'm an engineer. I'm trained to question inputs, question assumptions, question the sensor reading, question whether the whole system is lying to me.

Sometimes that's a strength. Sometimes it's just denial with better vocabulary.

The first cath was the beginning of the "known issue" phase. A thing you file away. A thing you put on the shelf next to dental checkups, oil changes, and "I really should start eating better." It's not that you ignore it completely. It's that you don't reorganize your life around it. You don't want to be the guy who talks about his heart all the time. You don't want to be fragile. You don't want the label.

Even as a kid, there were tells. During sports physicals—Little League, then school sports—doctors would take my blood pressure, pause, and call it "high normal." It was always verbal. Nobody put me on medication. I wasn't overweight. I was active. The unspoken assumption was: he's fine.

And yet I could feel how my system ran. I flushed easily. My face would go red during hard cardio well into my twenties. Not "I'm embarrassed" red—more like my baseline ran hot. It didn't mean I was sick. It meant there were patterns I didn't take seriously because I didn't have a reason to.

Then there was a moment early in my marriage that should have ended the debate. I was commuting from Midland to the Detroit area for work and something didn't feel right. Not dramatic pain—just wrong. I pulled off and went to a hospital. They took my blood pressure, then took it again. Then again. Multiple nurses, like they didn't trust what they were seeing.

It was high enough they weren't going to let me leave until they treated me. I stayed overnight.

That's the point I should have learned the lesson: this wasn't a one-off. The signs of hypertension had been there for years. I'd just gotten good at shoving them aside because I was young, busy, and functional. Functional is a dangerous standard.

And, if I'm honest, there was something else going on too: I didn't feel sick.

That's the trap. A lot of the worst problems don't announce themselves like a movie. They don't come with dramatic music and a collapse in a public place. They creep. They normalize. They let you keep functioning just enough that you can keep negotiating. You start using the absence of catastrophe as evidence that catastrophe isn't coming.

I had built a whole internal argument around that.

I hadn't dropped dead. I didn't have the

classic left-arm pain. I didn't have some clear, undeniable sign that would force me to stop everything and deal with it like a man dealing with something real. So I kept living like I had time. Like I could always tighten things up later.

Then the second cath happened, and the data got loud.

I remember trying to keep my engineer face on while the situation changed around me. You know that feeling when you're troubleshooting a system and you start out thinking it's going to be something minor—a bad connection, a flaky sensor, a little noise in the signal—and then you test one more thing and you realize the failure mode isn't "annoying." It's "catastrophic." The system isn't misbehaving. The system is headed for a hard stop.

The second cath was that moment.

The problem with being analytical is that you can always find a loophole. You can always find one more angle. One more story. One more "yeah, but."

Yeah, but I've been under stress and stress can do weird things.

Yeah, but I'm still doing my job.

Yeah, but I'm still walking around.

Yeah, but my cholesterol isn't terrible.

Yeah, but it's hereditary and they've been watching it.

Yeah, but I'm not in constant pain.

Yeah, but…

At some point you have to face the part that's

hard to admit: the "yeah, but" isn't logic. It's fear trying to buy time.

I don't say that as a moral lesson. I say it because it's what happened in my head. The second cath put a spotlight on the reality I'd been dancing around: I wasn't playing craps. I was playing Russian roulette. And the fact that I'd gotten away with it for a while wasn't proof that it was safe. It was proof that I'd been lucky.

Luck is not a plan.

When people say "open-heart surgery," it sounds like one big moment, like a single event. It isn't. It's a chain reaction. It's appointments, tests, conversations, waiting, and your brain trying to digest information that doesn't fit into your self-image.

Because here's the thing: I didn't walk around thinking of myself as someone who was going to need his chest opened. I didn't see myself that way. I had stress, sure. I had a lifestyle that wasn't exactly a health documentary. I had habits. I had excuses. I had the usual guy stuff: work hard, push through, don't whine, don't make it a thing.

And then suddenly it was a thing.

The second cath didn't just give me a recommendation. It gave me a fork in the road where one path was "keep pretending" and the other path was "accept reality." The path I wanted was a third option: "do something that fixes it without changing my life."

That option doesn't exist.

There's a moment in problems like this where you realize the "system" has constraints you don't get to negotiate with. I can negotiate with vendors. I can negotiate with timelines. I can negotiate with my own laziness, which I'm very skilled at. I cannot negotiate with blood flow.

At some point the conversation becomes simple, even if your emotions make it complicated. The heart needs what the heart needs. The question becomes whether you want to handle it on purpose, or whether you want the universe to handle it for you at the worst possible time.

The first time I felt the reality of it wasn't in a cath lab. It was later, when I was alone with it. When the noise drops off and you can hear your own thoughts again. When the hard truth comes through: this is real, and you're not going to outsmart it.

That's when the surreal feeling starts creeping in, even before anyone wheels you anywhere.

You start noticing the small things. The way you look at your hands. The way you listen to your own heartbeat. The way time feels different when you realize you're not invincible and you never were. You start doing math you didn't ask to do. You start thinking about your kids. Your grandkids. The things you still haven't done. The things you assumed you'd get to when you finally had the time.

You start realizing that "later" might not show up the way you think it will.

I'm not going to pretend I handled all of this like some stoic warrior. I had moments of clarity and moments of denial. I had moments where I felt calm and moments where I felt pissed off. I had moments where I told myself I was fine and moments where I knew I was not.

What I did have, consistently, was the need to understand. That's my version of control. If I can understand the system, I can at least face the failure honestly. If I can see the variables, I can stop lying to myself about what I'm doing.

That became my first real step toward recovery, and it happened before surgery ever did.

The second cath ended the debate. And even then, I tried to argue because I wanted the old story to be true: that I could keep living the same way and somehow outrun the consequences. The part of me that prides itself on being rational was still trying to negotiate with reality.

Reality didn't care.

Reality was simple: I had a problem that wasn't going to fix itself, and it had reached the point where the fix was going to be invasive, major, and unmistakable.

When the decision was made, everything shifted. Time compressed. The world kept moving like normal, and at the same time, my world narrowed down to a single point: there's a date on the calendar now where someone is going to open my chest and re-route blood around blockages that could kill me.

That sentence still sounds insane when I write it.

But it was my sentence.

And once it's your sentence, you start learning something fast: you can't think your way out of it. You can only go through it.

So that's what I did.

Next comes the lead-up—the mental game, the logistics, the strange calm that shows up at the worst possible times, and the moment where you realize you're not driving anymore.

You're being wheeled.

And that's where the surreal really starts.

THREE

System Overload
_____

To understand how I ended up staring at the ceiling before dawn on January 19th, we have to rewind to the summer before.

It started on a tennis court.

I was playing with my friend Chris. Nice summer day. Nothing unusual. I had played tennis in high school and in summer rec leagues in my twenties, though I hadn't kept up with it over the years. Earlier that same year, I'd played with another friend and felt fine. Not great—I was out of shape and knew it—but fine.

This was different.

We hadn't been playing long and I was already gassed. Out of breath. Fatigued in a way that didn't match the effort. We paused and tried to keep going, but I couldn't sustain it. I wasn't getting my ass kicked. I just couldn't keep up with simple shots. Rallies I should have been able to handle had me bent over, hands on knees, sucking air.

Here's the thing: Chris is about nine years older than me. And he was doing just fine.

I couldn't blame age. I couldn't blame the heat. A man in his sixties was outlasting me on a casual summer afternoon.

So I did what people do when the first warning light comes on. I found an explanation that let me keep moving.

Out of shape. Busy life. Too much weight. Pick your excuse.

Tennis is a sport you can play while out of shape. You adjust. You let balls go. You survive.

But I couldn't even do that.

I moved on and didn't think much of it.

Then came the lawn.

Typical midsummer Michigan day. Hot. Humid. The kind of air that feels like you're breathing through a wet wool blanket. I was in my backyard, push-mowing.

I wasn't a fragile man. Six feet tall. About 250 pounds. Overweight, sure, but I carried it like someone once active who had slowly transitioned into a desk jockey. Underneath it, I was still strong. I did projects. Handyman work. Hauled things around without asking for help.

But that day, the machine wasn't running right.

I didn't clutch my chest. I didn't collapse. I didn't have the Hollywood heart attack scene where the music swells and the screen fades to black.

I just felt… tired.

Not normal tired. Not "drink some water and keep going" tired. It was systemic. My chest felt tight, but not painful. Like an engine being starved of fuel. I was asking my body for horsepower, and the throttle wasn't responding.

I stopped the mower, wiped the sweat off my forehead, and drank water.

You're just out of shape, I told myself. It's ninety degrees. You're in your fifties. You're carrying too much weight. Of course you're tired.

As a process control engineer, I look at inputs and outputs. I looked at the inputs: heat + humidity + weight + exertion. The output: fatigue. The math checked out. Logical conclusion.

I was wrong.

In engineering terms, it was a false negative. I accepted the "normal" explanation because it was convenient. Because it let me keep doing what I'd been doing.

What I didn't know then is what I learned later: this wasn't "out of shape." This was my heart asking for oxygen it couldn't get fast enough. The pump was working, but the plumbing was compromised. The system was being starved under load.

But in the moment, I blamed the heat. I blamed the extra pounds. I blamed everything except the thing that mattered.

I'd been giving the medical world the runaround for years. I was a terrible patient. Hypertensive since I was young—during sports physicals, doctors called it "high normal." Later in life, it finally got a real label, and I was put on blood pressure medication, which I took grudgingly.

Then came cholesterol, statins, and the usual warnings. Years earlier, a heart cath had shown blockages. "We'll watch them," they said, and I got a prescription.

I hate pills. I'm forgetful if they aren't right in front of me. And frankly, I wasn't disciplined. I'd heard enough stories about side effects to give myself permission to become an expert in rationalization.

So I ignored maintenance warnings. I ignored the check-engine light.

I might have kept ignoring it until something catastrophic forced the issue, if not for my wife.

She's a seasoned ER nurse. She watched me come inside that day, sweaty and breathing heavier than I should have been for a basic lawn job. I mentioned the tightness. I mentioned the fatigue. I may have mentioned the tennis match, though honestly I don't remember trying to make it a big deal.

She didn't look at the heat or the humidity. She looked at the patient.

And she let me know that it was time to see a doctor, no more excuses.

And then she said it the way only an ER nurse can say it—half blunt, half protective, all truth. Loosely quoting her: she wasn't interested in wiping drool off my chin because I ignored this long enough to have a stroke. In other words: take care of your business now, while you still can.

So I did. I made the appointment. I got the referral. On paper, I did the right things.

Then I did the other thing I'm great at.

I kicked the can down the road.

The cath got scheduled. Then rescheduled. Then pushed. I told myself I was busy. Work, travel, life—pick your excuse. It didn't feel urgent because I wasn't in the kind of pain people think they're supposed to be in.

By the time the holidays rolled around, it still wasn't done.

Then right after the first of the year, the cath finally happened.

And that day, everything changed.

Looking back, I was a dumbass.

I was walking around with a system that wasn't getting the flow it needed, still doing normal things, still telling myself I was fine, still assuming I had time.

That's not toughness. That's denial dressed up as strength.

I didn't know I was walking into a diagnostic process that would uncover a system on the verge of catastrophic failure.

I just knew something felt off.

And "off" is the most dangerous symptom there is, because it's easy to explain away.

Until it isn't.

FOUR

The Widowmaker

The path to the operating table is rarely a straight line. It's usually a series of referrals, scheduling conflicts, and waiting rooms.

In my case, it started in the summer.

My primary care doctor—she listened to my symptoms and looked at my history—knew enough to take it seriously. I'd been hypertensive since I was young, but my labs were confusing. I was pushing into the pre-diabetic A1c range, but I wasn't diabetic. My cholesterol wasn't perfect, but it wasn't screaming "imminent death" either. It turns out you can't outrun bad genetics.

Usually, the next step in the flowchart is a stress test. They put you on a treadmill, hook you up to an EKG, and make you run the Bruce Protocol until your heart rate hits a target.

But I have a shitty knee. Years of wear and tear meant that in previous attempts, I'd stop because of joint pain long before my heart gave out. My doctor knew it. She decided to skip the treadmill charade and ordered a heart catheterization.

Here's where the story stops being about medicine and starts being about me.

It was scheduled pretty quickly. The referral was handled. The plan was in motion.

And then I delayed.

I rescheduled. I had conflicts. Work. Life. The same excuses I used everywhere else. The symptoms weren't dramatic, so it didn't feel urgent. I kept living like I had time.

Then the calendar rolled toward the holidays, and the delays stacked up. On top of my own procrastination, the cardiologist who would perform the cath wasn't available until right around the first of the year.

By then, I had talked myself into believing the most comfortable version of the story.

I felt fine. I was still doing handyman work. I was still riding my Peloton. I was ignoring the problem with the confidence of a man who thinks he knows better.

On a cold day in early January, I finally went in for the cath.

I'd had a heart cath before. Years earlier, they found two blockages—around fifty percent. Back then the strategy was watch and wait. I assumed this would be the same. Maybe they'd find a seventy percent blockage. Maybe they'd pop in a stent, I'd take a few days off, and I'd be back to work.

I woke up from sedation to see the cardiologist standing over me.

She didn't look like someone who had just placed a routine stent. She looked like someone who had just seen a ghost.

"Mr. Cummer," she said. "You have four blockages."

I blinked, trying to clear the fog. "Four?"

"Your Left Anterior Descending artery—the LAD—is ninety-nine percent blocked."

The LAD has another name in the medical world: the Widowmaker.

I lay there, processing the data. Ninety-nine percent blocked. That is a flow restriction that should have shut down the plant. One percent flow shouldn't support life, let alone a man who mows his lawn and rides a stationary bike.

"How am I not dead?" I asked.

Later, the surgeon would tell me something I still think about: my body had grown its own detours.

It turns out my system had recognized the starvation and built collateral flow—smaller pathways that kept blood moving around the worst blockage. A biological workaround. A temporary patch. The application stayed online without ever sending me a push notification that critical maintenance was happening in the background.

But the system was overloaded. I was circulating blood, but not enough oxygenated blood under load. I was running the engine on fumes.

The cardiologist explained that because of the number and location of the blockages, stents were off the table. This wasn't a clean little plumbing job. I needed open-heart surgery.

She told me not to exert myself.

My brain immediately went to work looking for the loophole.

"Well, I have a Peloton," I said. "I can still use that though, right?"

I wasn't joking. I was reasoning. The Peloton was exercise, sure, but it felt controlled. I could set the pace. I could control the resistance. It seemed manageable.

This is an engineer talking to a cardiologist, trying to logic my way into doing what I wanted. I'd been fine so far, hadn't I? I hadn't dropped dead yet. Surely there was room to negotiate.

Her eyes nearly popped out of her head. I saw genuine terror on her face. She looked like she was afraid to let me get off the table, let alone climb onto a bike.

"No," she said. "Absolutely not."

I didn't fully grasp it then. I was still operating like a man who had time, who had options. I didn't understand that I was one heartbeat away from a pipe bursting, and the only reason I was still alive was because my body had quietly built a detour around the wreckage.

I wasn't negotiating from a position of strength. I was a dead man asking for permission to exercise.

My wife took the news differently. She didn't

negotiate. She went into ER nurse mode. She absorbed the data, assessed the threat, and locked it down.

A few days later, we sat in the office of the heart surgeon.

He was warm and confident—the kind of guy who didn't need to bluster because he knew exactly what he was doing. He pulled up the video of my heart catheterization on a monitor.

For a moment, I stopped being a patient and went back to being an automation engineer. I've spent a lifetime building HMIs and staring at GUIs. I know what data looks like. I know how to read flow, pressure, and restriction.

Watching my own heart pump on that screen was fascinating. It was undeniable. If I claim to be logical—a chess player, a strategist, an engineer—I can't walk away from facts. The facts were pulsing right there in black and white.

"Here is the collateral flow," the surgeon pointed out. "And here is the blockage."

He paused, looking at the screen with something close to reverence. "The body is a beautiful machine, Mr. Cummer. It grew these pathways to save you."

I stared at the monitor and, for a moment, I allowed myself to nerd out.

If I were describing this as a system, my body looked like a modular application running on biological hardware. Somewhere in the background code, it detected a fault in the primary fuel line.

Plan A was simple: run as designed. That worked fine when I was younger, even with the hypertension. The code was clean enough. The pipes were clear enough.

But as the years passed and the blockage grew, the system threw an error. Instead of crashing the whole machine—a heart attack— the system executed Plan B. It initiated an internal patch. It grew collateral pathways and rerouted traffic through side streets because the highway was closing.

It fascinates me to this day. My body wrote its own workaround. It kept the application running, kept the user online, and didn't even send me an alert that the situation was critical.

But looking at that screen, I could also see the limit of the patch.

The workaround had held, but the demand was now exceeding the throughput. Internal repair was no longer enough.

We needed external intervention.

"You need a double bypass," the surgeon said, pulling me out of my analysis.

He explained that I needed surgery now, and that in a handful of years I might need a stent or two. He wasn't trying to scare me. He was treating me like an adult.

I heard him talking. I saw his lips moving. But there were moments where the sound just dropped out.

I was staring at the screen, and the word surreal finally clicked into place. People use that word all the time, but until you're sitting in a chair watching the mechanical failure of your own vital organ, you don't really know what it means. It felt like I was watching a movie about someone else.

I tried to snap back. I tried to regain control.

"Okay," I said, leaning forward. "I have some business conferences coming up next month. My company needs me. The work demands it. Can we schedule this for later in the spring? I can get my affairs in order, do the trips, and we can knock this out in March or April."

I was trying to negotiate with the data. I was trying to bargain with biology.

The surgeon smiled—kind, but firm. "Mr. Cummer," he said. "You will have plenty of conferences and Christmases ahead of you. But not if we wait."

Before I could push back, my wife stepped in. She'd been rattled since the cath lab—I knew she'd been making calls, ensuring we didn't leave without a plan—but now she was pure steel.

"Absolutely not," she said. "He is not going to any conferences. We are doing this now."

The surgeon nodded. "Two weeks," he said.

I slumped back in the chair.

For as long as I can remember, people have depended on me—my family, my colleagues, my people. I was the guy who kept the systems running. And now I was being benched. The game was going to continue, the world was going to keep spinning, and I was being forced to the sidelines.

I had walked into that office thinking I was indispensable.

I walked out realizing that if I wanted to be indispensable later, I had to survive the present.

FIVE

What I Was Told

(AND WHAT I ACTUALLY HEARD)

Let me clear something up.

People did tell me.

Doctors told me. Family told me. My spouse told me. Friends told me. Sometimes it was direct. Sometimes it was subtle. Sometimes it was said once. Sometimes it was said ten times.

I wasn't uninformed.

What I was—at times—was selective.

I had that "yeah, but me" thing. The quiet kind. Not the loud macho version. The version that sounds reasonable in your own head.

Yeah, but I'm still working.

Yeah, but I feel fine.

Yeah, but my cholesterol isn't that bad.

Yeah, but it's hereditary.

Yeah, but I'm not having left-arm pain.

Yeah, but…

On paper, those sound like data points. In reality, that's not logic. That's fear buying time.

"Yeah, but" is how you turn a legitimate warning light into background noise. Somebody says, "You should really get that checked out," and instead of hearing, "You might have a serious problem," you hear, "You're being offered an optional errand."

I told myself stories to make it easier to ignore things:

- I'm busy. I'll get to it.
- I'm not as bad as that guy.
- I'm tired because I work hard, not because anything's wrong.
- It's probably stress.

All technically possible. None of them guaranteed to be true. But in my head, they were comforting enough to win the argument—for a while.

And here's the other truth that nobody likes to admit because it ruins the neat story:

Genetics matter.

A lot.

I was predisposed to hypertension early. My system ran hot. I built plaque. That's the hand I was dealt. You can do a lot of things "right" and still end up in trouble. You can do a lot of things "wrong" and still get lucky.

That's not moral. That's biology and probability.

So I'm not going to preach at you like I found a magic formula.

Diet and exercise matter. Sleep matters. Stress matters. Meds matter when you need them. Doing the right things improves your odds.

But odds are not guarantees.

If you're looking for certainty, medicine can't give it to you. It can give you percentages, ranges, risk profiles. It can move you into a better column on the chart. It can't promise you a specific outcome.

Here's the framework that makes sense to me now—engineer-style.

Things you can control:

- Pay attention to symptoms instead of negotiating with them.
- Go to the appointments you schedule.
- Do the follow-ups instead of assuming "no news is good news."
- Take the meds you and your doctor decide you need, not just the ones you like.
- Move your body. Do the rehab. Rebuild the system.
- Get labs done when they're ordered instead of waiting until it's convenient.
- Tell your people what matters while you're still here to tell them.

Things you can't control:

- Your genetics.
- How fast something progresses in your body.
- Whether the timing works out cleanly.
- Whether a "routine procedure" gets complicated.
- Whether life throws a curveball you didn't earn.

The mistake I made wasn't that I didn't know what was recommended.

The mistake was acting like the recommendations were for other people.

Acting like I could negotiate with biology.

Acting like time was an unlimited resource.

When a doctor says, "We should keep an eye on that," what you want to hear is, "You're fine for now; don't worry about it." What they're actually saying is, "This could become a problem. Let's not lose track of it." I translated too many of those into permission slips.

Looking back, there were moments where I essentially said to my own body, "Yeah, I see your warning signs, but I've got a meeting." Or, "Yeah, that number's not great, but I've seen worse." That's not bravery. That's gambling.

So if you take one thing from this page, let it be this:

Do what improves your odds, and do it early.

Not because it guarantees anything.

Because it's the only move that makes sense when the alternative is rolling dice with a system you don't fully control.

No guarantees.

Still worth it.

SIX

The General

The diagnosis was in. The date was set. I had
two weeks.

Two weeks is a strange amount of time. It's
too short to live a lifetime, but too long to just
hold your breath. It's a purgatory where you
walk around as a free man, knowing you're
scheduled for execution—or at least scheduled to
be killed and brought back to life.

My reaction to stress has always been to
compartmentalize. I go into Command Mode. If
the leader panics, the troops panic. And I had a
lot of troops—my wife, my adult children, my
grandchildren.

So I decided to play the role of the General.

I walked around acting like it was no big
deal. Routine maintenance, I projected. The
Maytag Repair Man is going to swap out a few
hoses. Nothing to see here.

I smiled. I joked. I played Papa with the
grandkids—I'm keeping things normal while

inside my head a countdown clock was ticking. Fourteen days. Thirteen days.

I didn't want my grandchildren to have a core memory of Papa looking scared. I didn't want to add to the collective anxiety. So I kept it steady. I buried whatever I was feeling under layers of stoicism and dark humor.

"Well," I'd say to friends, "if I don't make it, at least I won't have to pay taxes this year." Or some other dumb line to distract people from knowing that I was actually nervous.

I laughed. They laughed—uncomfortably. That's my coping mechanism. If I can make a joke about it, it can't kill me.

A friend of mine—his dad is a doctor—was pretty cavalier about the whole thing.

"Bobby, don't worry about it," he said. "This happens all the time. It's routine. You'll get through it."

I appreciated that. It helped me stay level. But here's the thing: no matter how many people tell you it's routine, you don't know. You can't know. They're not the ones going under. The fact that they're standing there reassuring you instead of lying on the table themselves should tell you something.

People mean well. But their certainty can't become yours. You don't know until you're there.

My wife wasn't panicking either, but she was watching me closely. As we got closer to the surgery date, she seemed almost flabbergasted that I wasn't more rattled.

She didn't need me to fall apart. She just wanted to know I was taking it seriously. And I was—just not in a way that looked like fear.

The friction came to a head during the password talk.

That Christmas—just weeks before the surgery—she gave me a book called *WTF Is My Password*. The title says it all. She wanted me to write everything down. Account numbers, logins, credentials. The keys to our digital life.

"I don't even know how to get into our accounts if something happens to you," she said. "I need to know these things."

I understood the concern, but I wasn't worried about it.

"If anything happens," I told her, "Mitch will make sure you're taken care of. He's an attorney. He'll help you get into whatever you need."

I'd already solved the problem in my head. I had a network. I had people who could make things happen. The logistics were covered.

But looking back, I'm not sure logistics were what she was asking for.

She wasn't worried about lawyers and legal access. She wanted to be let in. She didn't want to feel like a stranger to her own life if I didn't come home.

I was solving an engineering problem. She was trying to connect.

It was simple stuff—bank account numbers, insurance papers, the Netflix login. Fortunately, we shared a PIN for the main bank card, but the rest of it? It was all in my head.

That exercise is yet one more surreal thing—documenting the keys to your life just in case you don't come back.

I didn't ask her if she was scared. I didn't tell her I was scared. I just organized the papers and moved on.

During those two weeks, I never really cracked. Not in front of family, not in private. I stayed in General mode the whole time. Some people might call that strength. Some might call it avoidance. I don't know which it was.

Maybe both.

What I do know is this: being told something is routine doesn't make it feel routine. You can read all the statistics. You can hear all the reassurances. But when it's your chest they're cutting open, when it's your heart they're stopping, the math doesn't comfort you.

You don't know until you're there.

And I was about to be there.

SEVEN

Go Time

_____

The drive to St. Mary's in Saginaw was dark. Pre-dawn, mid-January, Michigan winter. The kind of cold that seeps into the car before the heater can fight back.

My wife drove. At least, I think she did. Honestly, it's a blur. A lot of that morning is.

We chose St. Mary's because it was her hospital. She worked there—an ER nurse. She knew the hallways, the staff, the way things worked. Insurance probably played a role too, but more than anything, this was her turf.

Except now she wasn't showing up for a shift.

She was walking in as the wife of a cardiac surgery patient.

Same building. Completely different experience.

Walking into a hospital for a bypass isn't like walking in for a broken arm. You aren't walking toward a cure. You're walking toward a trauma that's necessary to save you.

They checked me in. Verified my identity. "Please state your name and date of birth." I answered. Robert Cummer. August 27, 1970. They matched me to their paperwork. I was the right guy.

Lucky me.

Then came the scale.

I stepped on. The number flashed. And immediately, the engineer in me woke up and chose violence.

Wait a minute, I thought. I'm wearing heavy winter shoes. Last time I was weighed, I was in slippers. Is this thing calibrated?

I stood there, moments away from having my chest opened, and I was genuinely annoyed about the data integrity of my weigh-in.

It was displacement. I couldn't control the blockage, so I fixated on the scale.

The pre-op room was cold and clinical. My wife was there with me at first. We talked, though I don't remember about what. Probably nothing important. Just filling the silence.

Then they told her she had to leave so they could prep me.

She said something. I said something back. And then she was gone.

That was the moment it got real.

My wife—the person who had been with me through all of this, who had pushed me to see the doctor, who had shut down my attempts to delay—was now on the other side of a door.

And I was alone with strangers who were about to open my chest.

She knew this hospital. She had walked these halls hundreds of times in scrubs, as the one providing care. Now she was on the other side, waiting to find out if her husband would survive.

I started talking. A lot.

When I get nervous, I become a chatterbox. I don't pace. I don't tremble. I talk. I make jokes (usually inappropriate). I fill the air with words so the silence can't get in.

A tech came in to prepare my body. In medical terms, "prepare" means removing anything that might catch fire or cause infection. In practical terms, it means you strip down and lie on a table that feels like a slab of ice.

I lay there—a middle-aged guy with a dad bod and notoriously dry skin—shivering in the cold room.

She produced a razor. No hot towel. No shaving cream. Just the dry scrape of steel against dry skin.

She shaved my chest, my legs, everywhere required. Efficient, impersonal, and excruciating.

I remember thinking: in some ways, this is going to be more painful than the actual surgery. At least during surgery, I'll be asleep. Here, I'm wide awake, naked, freezing, and being dry-shaved like a damn yak.

It was the ultimate stripping away of dignity. I wasn't a CTO or an engineer anymore. I wasn't a problem-solver or the guy people called when things went sideways. I was just a body being prepped for the assembly line.

Once I was scraped and gown-clad, the anesthesiologist arrived. He introduced himself and informed me that he'll be putting me to sleep.

I know that I made some sort of *genius, witty* joke that he'd never heard before in all his years of anesthesiology.

He assured me. Then he pushed the meds.

They wheeled me into the operating room. Cold. Sterile. Blindingly bright.

Holy shit. This is really happening.

I remember the surgical team introducing themselves. Saying hello to the surgeon. Voices telling me they were going to take care of me, that I was going to be okay.

They put the mask on me.

And my brain did what brains do when they're about to lose control. It started spinning up irrational questions—things I knew wouldn't happen, but couldn't stop wondering about anyway.

Is there enough gas? Will I be out fast enough before they start?

I trusted them. I knew they knew what they were doing. But you can't always stop the mind from racing when you're lying there, watching the ceiling, knowing what comes next.

I closed my eyes.

And then I opened them.

They were done.

I think it was nearly five hours of surgery and recovery. But just a blink for me.

I was in post-Op. A tube was down my throat. And my first thought, through the fog, was simple.

No shit.

I made it.

EIGHT

Reboot

The first face I saw was my surgeon.

"Hello, Robert. You did just fine."

Simple words. But in that moment, they meant everything.

They moved me to a post-surgical room and notified my wife that I was out. Eventually, they wheeled me into the Cardiac Care Unit. It was quiet. Lights dim. The kind of stillness that tells you this is where they put people who just had their chests cracked open.

I had a tube down my throat.

Most people panic when they wake up intubated. They gag. They fight it. But my lungs were already online. The system was booting up faster than they expected. I opened my eyes and immediately tried to speak.

It's over. I made it.

They realized I was awake—really awake—and moved fast. They extubated me right there.

I coughed, took a breath of cold, sharp air, and looked down.

There were drainage tubes snaking out of my chest. Three of them—thick, industrial hoses that felt like they were anchored somewhere deep inside me. There was also a pacing wire in place in case they needed to nudge my heart back into rhythm. And underneath it all, I felt the tightness.

The piano wire.

My sternum had been split and wired back together. I wasn't just flesh and bone anymore. I was reinforced structure.

And then there were my legs.

I'd gone in thinking "heart surgery" meant my chest. I woke up realizing it's a whole-body job. I had incisions in both calves—because one of the standard conduits for bypass is a leg vein, most often the great saphenous vein that runs up the inside of your leg. They don't just take a little snippet. They have to free a usable length of vessel and deal with all the little branch connections along the way.

My primary care doctor explained it to me later in plain English, and it finally clicked. He told me that earlier in his career, harvesting those veins used to be part of his job. The vein has side branches, and those branches have to be ligated—tied off or clipped—so the vessel can be removed cleanly and repurposed as a graft. In older-style harvesting, that could mean longer incisions up the leg because you're basically doing careful plumbing work under the skin. The leg isn't a side note. It's a second procedure running in parallel with the main one.

And yes—the "mammary" part.

I used to describe it as "they took a vein from my left breast," because that's how it landed in my head at the time: chest, left side, something harvested. What I understand now is that in many bypass surgeries they use the left internal mammary artery—also called the internal thoracic artery—which runs along the inside of the chest wall behind the sternum. It's an artery, not a vein, and it's commonly used as a graft to the LAD. In other words: part of my bypass wasn't borrowed from my leg at all—it was re-routed from inside my own ribcage.

My chest was covered in surgical glue and staples. My calves were sutured—though not well, in my opinion. I still have scars today. They've faded, but they're there. Permanent reminders.

The doctor came in. Then my wife. She sat with me. I don't remember exactly what she said, but she was there.

That was enough.

I wanted out of there as fast as they would let me go. Not "Tuesday." Not "five days." Just: get me the hell out of this place. If they'd cleared me sooner, I would've left sooner. Tuesday was just the day the paperwork finally matched my attitude.

They didn't give me any indication early release was realistic. You don't just check out of a cardiac ICU because you're motivated. You have to earn your release. You have to prove you aren't a liability.

The first night was a disaster.

I'm a shallow breather by nature. Sometimes I have long pauses between breaths—my idle speed is just set low. But the monitors didn't like my idle speed. Every time I drifted off, my oxygen dipped below their threshold and the alarms screamed.

BEEP. BEEP. BEEP.

Nurses would rush in, waking me up to "keep me on track." It was torture by sensor. I lay there exhausted, wired shut, listening to machines panic about a problem I didn't feel.

Then there was the food. Initially, they put me on a restricted diabetic diet—standard protocol for cardiac patients. It was cardboard. Then the blood work came back.

My A1C was 5.2.

For a guy my size, that number felt like a trophy. It proved my metabolism wasn't broken—just my arteries. The diet restriction was lifted. Small victories.

To get out, I had to pass their tests. Prove my lungs worked. Prove I could manage pain. Prove I could move.

Getting out of that bed the first time was an education in agony.

The drainage tubes pulled with every movement. I couldn't get comfortable in the chair—they were too long, too awkward, and everything hurt. But I got into the chair anyway. Then I got onto my feet.

I started walking.

At first, they only wanted me to go a short distance. But I started pacing the hallways. Tubes swaying, chest aching, determined to prove the system was operational.

A physician's assistant pulled me aside later. He told me the staff had been watching me.

"You had one of the most difficult surgeries we offer here," he said. "And the staff can see that you're determined. You're doing everything you can to move, to get better. There are patients here with less severe injuries who won't even get out of bed. You've been an example."

I appreciated that. But I wasn't trying to be an example. I just had a drive. A simple equation in my head: I'm going to do this. I'm going to get home. And to get home, I have to prove I'm ready.

Not forcing my body. Not being reckless. Just refusing to wait for recovery to happen to me.

On Sunday, they pulled the tubes.

The clinician who did it was brisk. No gentleness. No easing into it. She told me to exhale and yanked them out. The drainage tubes. The wire. All of it.

It hurt like hell. Honestly, I didn't have a very nice opinion of that clinician immediately afterwards; even one of the techs that had been helping me since arrival in the Cardia Care Unit had a look on his face that was one of shock! But when they were gone, I felt so much better. Like the anchors had been cut and I could finally move.

On Saturday, my friend Bruce came to visit.

He drove through a Michigan winter snowstorm to see me. We had only known each other a couple of years, but we had a connection and he was such a good dude. He walked into my room, shook off the snow, and stopped dead.

I was sitting up in the chair. Alert. Ready to leave.

"I don't believe it," he said.

Bruce sat down and shared his own story. He'd undergone heart surgery a year prior. But unlike me, he hadn't bounced back. He showed me photos on his phone—his hands and legs swollen with fluid, his body failing to reboot.

Bruce had a weak ejection fraction. His pump was tired.

That was the moment it hit me. I had shitty genetics when it came to plumbing—my arteries were a mess. But I'd been gifted something else. My heart muscle itself was strong. The pump was a thoroughbred.

Bruce came to support me. Instead, he taught me how lucky I was.

Sadly, Bruce died the following year from heart related issues. I think of him often.

Standing there in that hospital room with my chest wired shut and my calves stitched up, I looked at him and felt something shift—deep gratitude, vibrating under the surface.

I had survived the one percent. I had survived the ninety-nine percent blockage. And I was walking.

Later, I found out who had been in the waiting room while I was on the table. I really didn't know there was a communication network between family and friends operating behind the scenes. I didn't know any of that while I was under. I just knew I had to make it.

And I did.

Over the course of the next several days I did everything I could possibly do to prove to the staff that I was ready for discharge. Two words were burned into my brain: determination and perseverance. Breathing exercises and walking as much as they'd let me.

On Tuesday, they cut me loose.

The paperwork took forever—it always does. But I thanked the staff before I left. They had been good to me. Kind, helpful, encouraging.

The ride home was nerve-racking. Every bump in the road shot through my chest. Even in a Tahoe with good suspension, I felt everything. My sternum felt like it was floating, held together by wire, and I was terrified it wouldn't heal straight. I sat rigid, careful with every movement, worried about shifting side to side.

My wife drove carefully. But there's no way to make a road smooth when your chest has been split open.

When we pulled up to the house, I stepped down slowly. Carefully.

I walked inside.

My recliner was waiting for me in the living room. That was my new bed. For a while, I wasn't allowed to sleep flat—only reclined. My wife took my vitals. There was some edema in my legs, some pitting in my calves. She checked my blood pressure, made sure I had my meds, and did what she could to make me comfortable.

I was home.

Five days from surgery to my own living room. The doctors didn't think it was possible. But I made it.

Part One was over.

One more thing, for the record: this is how I remember it.

I haven't asked anyone else to fill in blanks or validate details, and I did that on purpose. By the time you're reading this, it will have been three years (or more) since the surgery happened. Memory isn't a transcript. It's a lens. There may be differences in how other people remember pieces of it, but this is my story, through my eyes, the way time stored it.

That matters, because recovery isn't only physical. It's also how you make meaning out of what happened to you.

Surgery is an event. Recovery is a process.

Part I was the event—how it unfolded, and how it hit me.

Part II is the process: the small realities, the mental traps, and the few things that actually helped.

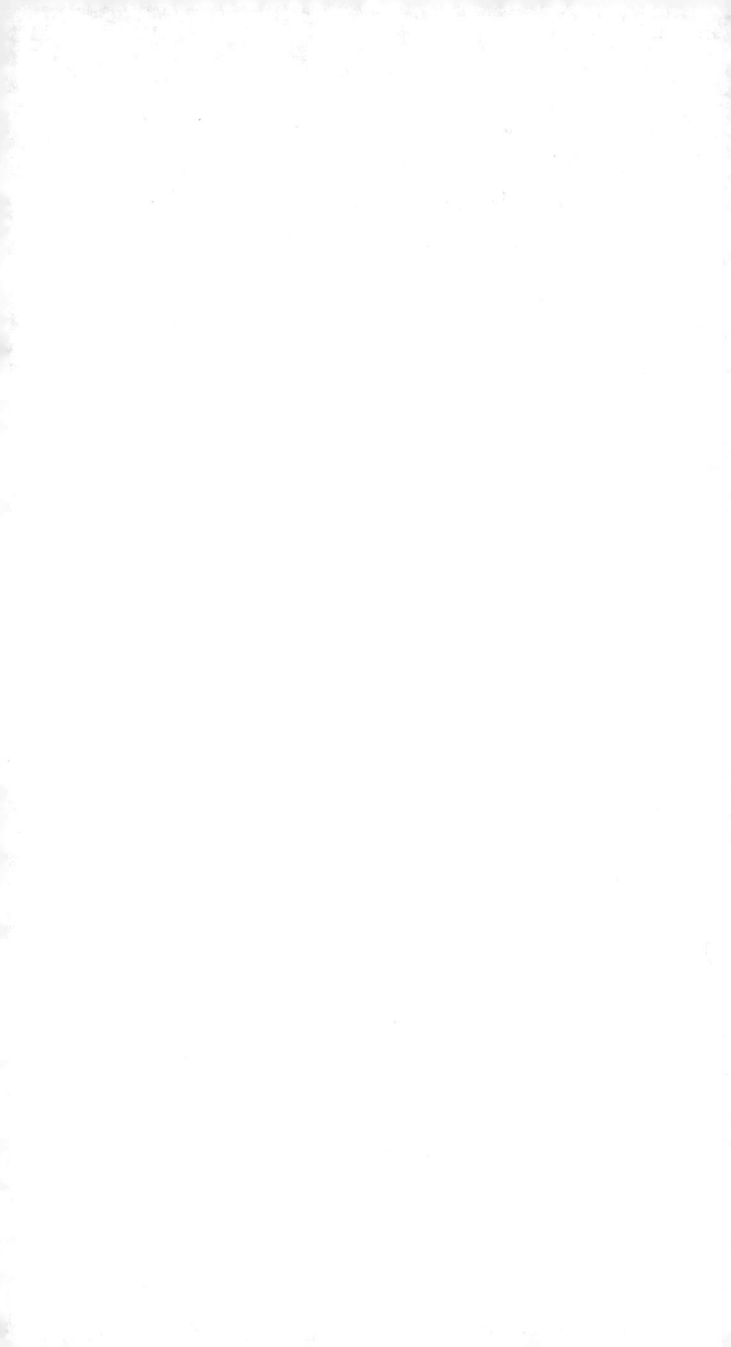

PART II
Work the Problem

I wish I could tell you there's a clean finish line. There isn't.

Surgery is a moment in time. Recovery is the part that keeps showing up when you think the story is over.

The incision closes. The scar settles. Everyone else exhales. You get the "you look great" comments. And inside you're thinking, *Okay… so why do I still feel off?*

This is the part nobody really maps for you —not because people don't care, but because it's messy and personal and hard to put into words.

So I'm going to put it into words the only way I know how: like troubleshooting. What failed. What helped. What didn't. What I see now.

NINE

What I See Now

Recently, I listened to a public figure I've followed for years—a cartoonist, a writer, a guy who's always been blunt—talk about the fact that he's exhausted the treatment options for his cancer. He said it the way he says everything: pragmatically. No melodrama. Just the reality, delivered straight.

He's received an outpouring of love and support from people all over the world. I think it's because he's been authentic. From his work to his worst days, he's just been himself. That matters. People respond to real.

Since my surgery, I've tried to figure out how to put my own view of life into words. It's harder than it sounds. The surgery and the immediate aftermath didn't depress me—other personal and professional events did that later. But getting through that operating room, getting off that table, changed my internal settings.

It gave me a renewed view of life. An appreciation I didn't have before.

The most important people in my world are my family and my closest friends. People who have been authentic with me. My tribe—not just by blood, but by choice. That's how I think about it now. Roots wide and deep.

There were people who stopped by the house just to sit with me. Some were local. Others drove a half hour, an hour, two hours, just to check in and burn a chunk of their day on a guy in a recliner. They didn't act like it was a big deal. No speeches. No fanfare. They just showed up.

It made me think about how selfish I'd been at times. How many times I'd told myself I was "too busy" to make that same kind of drive for somebody else. Meanwhile, here were people rearranging their schedules to come watch bad TV with me and ask how I was doing.

You learn to pay attention to that. Never forget the people who choose to spend their time on you. They could be anywhere, doing anything, and they decide to be in your living room instead. Why? Maybe that's just who they are. Maybe it's because of a hundred small moments you shared over the years. Either way, it's a quiet reminder that there are good people in the world —and that you actually need them more than you thought.

Some of the visitors were expected: close family, lifelong friends. Some were surprises. A guy you haven't seen in a while who suddenly appears with a casserole. Somebody's spouse who brings over a family soup recipe "because protein helps healing". A friend who doesn't cook, but shows up with takeout and sits there so you have someone to talk to.

Then there were the gifts that forced me to look at the future.

My cousin Stephanie sent a heart-healthy cookbook. It wasn't a generic "get well soon" gesture; it was an instruction manual for the new operating system. While others were bringing comfort food—which I appreciated—that book sat on the counter reminding me that the days of ignoring the fuel mixture were over.

Her sister, my cousin Liz, sent a plant. But not flowers. Flowers are temporary; they die in a week. Liz sent a Lucky Bamboo—which isn't actually bamboo, but a tough little survivor that grows in just water and rocks.

The stalks were trained into the shape of hearts. Literally twisted and bent, but still green.It didn't ask to be coddled. It just needed a little light and the occasional drink. I'm looking at it right now. It is the three-year anniversary of my surgery, and that

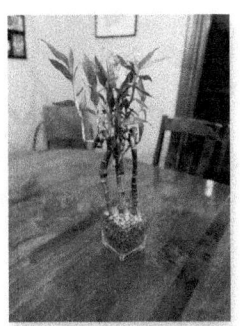

Day 1

plant is still sitting there, growing and stubborn.

We both made it.

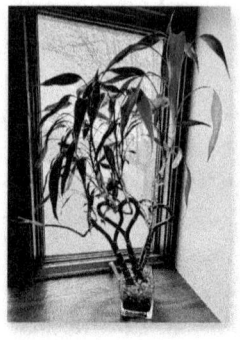

3 years later

"How are you feeling?" becomes the standard opener. You don't give the same answer to everyone. There are a few people you can be brutally honest with: "Today sucks. I hurt. I'm tired of this chair". With others, you keep it lighter. They're still asking because they care, but you can feel the difference between polite concern and the kind of curiosity that has a little morbid edge to it—*What does it actually feel like to have your chest opened and rewired?*

Even the phone calls and messages mattered. Texts, emails, social media comments—things that usually feel like background noise suddenly land differently. Social media can be a disaster most days, but in that season, it turned into a signal boost of encouragement. Old coworkers, distant relatives, people I hadn't talked to in years sent little notes: thinking of you, praying for you, pulling for you.

It didn't fix the pain, but it changed the weather in my head.

All of that forced me to see something I'd been blind to: you don't always know how important you are to people. Sometimes it isn't about some grand gesture you made. It's that you showed up for them once, or you shared a season of life together, or you made them laugh on a hard day. And when it's your turn on the table—or your turn in the recliner—they remember.

Those are your people. That's your tribe. They don't have to be with you every day, shoulder-to-shoulder. They can be scattered across towns and states and time zones. But when things break, they close ranks.

Maybe that's why I don't get so spun up about politics anymore. I still lean toward one side more than the other, but I don't get flipped out like I used to. It's all a big show, and I'm not willing to donate my peace of mind to it.

I'm still attached to my sports teams, but not like before. The outcomes don't wreck me the way they once did. I still care, but it doesn't feel like life or death—because now I've been close enough to actual life and death to know the difference.

Recently, I lost one of my best friends. His name was Craig. He died just before his 55th birthday. Supposedly natural causes—which probably means a heart attack in his sleep. No foul play. Just gone.

Craig was the only person I ever lived with outside of a significant other. We shared a college dorm. An apartment. A lot of years. A lot of memories. He was a genuine, good person.

I found out during a Lions game. They lost that day. I remember thinking, of all the times for the world to deliver bad news, it picked a Sunday afternoon where I'm already braced for disappointment. The difference was this wasn't a game. This was permanent.

Sometimes Craig would text me out of nowhere: "Go Lions." That was it. Sometimes he would call randomly in the middle of the day just to say, "I love you, see you," and hang up. He didn't get to see his 55th birthday. He didn't get to see my book released. *Dark Recipe* came out on what would have been his birthday. He died the Sunday before. A week short.

Maybe he knows. Maybe he sees it. Maybe he's watching me write about him right now.

I don't have the answer. I don't mock anyone who believes he does. I just don't know what's out there. What I do know is this: I smell things differently now. I notice things I never noticed before. I find myself stopping to take photos of frozen twigs on a tree. Rocks with ice on them. Little scenes frozen in time. Quiet, temporary, and somehow beautiful.

I can't stand the cold—I really can't—but I recognize beauty when I see it now. I stop. I appreciate it. And I wonder how I missed it before.

I also notice something else now: the way we all pretend we're not scared. We'll talk about "odds" and "routines" and "good hands," because that's what people do when they don't have control. We use language like armor. We tell ourselves we're being rational. We tell ourselves we're being strong. We tell ourselves we're being brave.

But sometimes the bravest thing you can do is admit what you're actually feeling. Because fear doesn't mean you're weak. Fear means you understand the stakes. Fear means you're paying attention.

And if you're staring at a calendar date where someone is going to stop your heart and restart it, fear is a sane response.

If you're there now—if you've got that date circled, if you're lying awake at three in the morning doing math you didn't ask to do— here's what I wish someone had told me before I walked into St. Mary's:

It's okay to be scared.

TEN

It's Okay to Be Scared (Or Just Numb)

Let me correct something. I've used the word "scared," but looking back, that's not exactly right.

I wasn't shaking in a corner. I wasn't crying.

I was in a fog.

That two-week waiting period is a fucked-up time. You're walking around the grocery store, or sitting at work, or watching TV, and everything looks normal—but it feels like you're watching it through thick glass. You know a train is coming, you know the arrival time, and you're just standing on the tracks waiting for it.

Time moves strangely. Some hours crawl. Some days disappear. You catch yourself staring at a spreadsheet, or a TV show, or a face in front of you, and you realize you haven't heard a word in the last five minutes. You read the same paragraph three times. You stand in the kitchen and forget why you walked in there. It's not dramatic.

It's just like your brain is running on a half-second delay.

Sleep gets weird too. You fall asleep in front of the TV, then bolt awake at three in the morning with your heart pounding—not because anything is happening, but because your mind finally found a quiet moment to spin. You lie there in the dark doing math you don't want to do: success rates, ages, birthdays, things you've done, things you haven't done yet. You're too tired to think clearly and too wired to rest.

And then there are the people.

Everyone who knows you wants to help. They love you. They care. But it gets weird for everyone.

They ask, "How are you doing?"

It's the most loaded question in the world. What are you supposed to say? "Well, I'm waiting for someone to saw my sternum in half." No. You can't say that. It makes them uncomfortable. It makes you sound ungrateful for their optimism.

So you say, "I'm hanging in there. Ready to get it over with."

Then they give you the reassurance.

"You're going to be okay."

"My uncle had this, he's fine."

"You've got this."

They say it because they don't know what else to say. They feel helpless, so they offer certainty. They want to wrap you in the story where everything works out. They're trying to make you feel better, but half the time, you end up comforting them. You end up nodding and smiling and acting confident just to relieve the tension in the room.

It's exhausting.

You're carrying the weight of the surgery, and you're also carrying the weight of making sure everyone around you is okay with it.

Meanwhile, your mind does what minds do when there's a hard line on the calendar: it wanders.

I have to admit I did a little daydreaming in that waiting period. My thoughts bounced between two channels: What is life going to look like after heart surgery? and What if the lights really do turn off? What happens if I don't wake up?

For a long time, I've considered myself agnostic, even if I didn't always use that word. That started with the early deaths in my family. My mom's fraternal twin brother died in 1987. She died in 1989, two days before my nineteenth birthday. They were thirty-seven and thirty-nine years old.

They didn't die in freak accidents. They died from lifestyle. Poor choices. Poor decisions. Effectively, they drank themselves to death.

At the time, I was living with my grandparents. They were raising me. Within two years, they lost both of their children.

I watched my grandmother, Betty, dive into religion and support groups. She got confirmed

Lutheran. The pastor would come to the house to meet with her and my grandfather, Robert. Sometimes I was home; sometimes I wasn't. I knew when the pastor was there, but I mostly stayed out of the way. My grandfather kept to himself too. He didn't sit in on the visits. He grieved differently, more internally, or maybe he didn't know what to do with a God who allowed both his kids to die before forty.

I also watched them leave my uncle's bedroom exactly the way he left it for a long time. Years. Even after my mom died, that room stayed frozen—clothes in drawers, things on shelves, like he might walk back in any minute. The door was there. The room was there. The person wasn't.

Try processing that as a teenager.

I had a hard time understanding how two good people could lose both of their children so young. How that fit into any kind of plan. How God—if there was one—could sign off on that. I didn't get any satisfying answers. So I did the only honest thing I could do: I admitted I didn't know.

I wasn't a full-on atheist. I wasn't a committed believer either. I was undecided. I had been baptized Episcopalian. I went to Christmas Eve services sometimes. I had friends who were Christian, Catholic, Lutheran, all of it. I tagged along now and then. But if I'm honest, I was just going with the flow, not building a belief system.

Fast-forward to the weeks before surgery, and those old questions came back, only louder.

Shit. Am I going to meet my Maker? Or is it just darkness? Is there something on the other side of this, or is this it? Did I check the right boxes? Did I even understand what the boxes were?

This isn't meant to be offensive to anyone reading this who is deeply religious. I'm not taking shots at your faith. I'm just telling you what ran through my head. I'm not claiming to have the answers. I'm not judging yours. I'm just being honest and real about where I was.

On paper, my life looked good. I had a beautiful family. A home I was proud of. Work I cared about. A wife and children I loved. Part of me hoped that meant I'd done enough of the "right things" to get past the pearly gates—if there are pearly gates. I never said that out loud. I internalized it. As smart as I'm perceived to be by some people—engineer, problem-solver, data guy—I didn't know everything. So I kept my mouth shut and let the questions rattle around in my own head.

That's one of the strangest parts of the waiting period: the outside world sees you as the brave patient marching toward surgery, while the inside of your head is a mix of grocery lists, hospital instructions, and late-night theology you're not sure you believe.

I've heard some people say they're prepared. That they're fully at peace with themselves and with life. Maybe they are. I wasn't there. I just knew I had more to do. More I wanted to build and write and share with my people. I wasn't ready to set it down yet. I wasn't done being a dad, a grandfather, a friend. I wasn't done being me.

So yes, in that sense, I was scared. Not horror-movie scared. Not curled-up-in-a-ball scared. But aware. Aware that I might not get as many tomorrows as I'd been casually assuming. Aware that the universe doesn't owe me a full set of retirement years just because I had plans.

And all of that is happening while you're trying to answer, "How are you doing?" in a way that doesn't freak anyone out.

Here's what I want you to hear if you're in that window now:

If you feel like you're moving in slow motion while the rest of the world is on fast forward—that's normal.

If you feel numb instead of terrified—that's normal.

If you're quietly imagining both versions of the future—the one where you walk out of the hospital and the one where you don't—that's normal.

If you get annoyed when people tell you "It's going to be fine" because they aren't the ones putting on the gown—that's normal too.

You don't have to perform for anyone. You don't have to be the stoic warrior, and you don't have to be the sobbing wreck. You can just be the person in the fog, doing the best you can to put one day after the other.

That fog is your brain trying to protect you. It's a buffer. It lets you function enough to show up when it's time without collapsing under the weight of every possible outcome.

So if you're in that waiting period right now, and you feel detached from your own life, don't beat yourself up. You don't need to force an emotion you don't feel, or fake certainty you don't have.

You just have to get through the days.

Let them ask. Nod your head. Say thanks. Do what you need to do to get your body and your paperwork where they're supposed to be.

And when the day comes, walk in with whatever you've got—fear, questions, fog and all.

The courage isn't in never being scared. The courage is in showing up anyway.

ELEVEN

Fuck My Life, Keep Going

Sometime after my surgery, I decided to become a private pilot.

Not for a career. Not to impress anybody. This was one of those things I needed to do for myself. I'd wanted to fly since high school—since seeing Top Gun and watching jets carve the sky like it was nothing. Life got in the way. I told myself I'd get to it "someday," and someday kept moving.

Heart surgery has a way of dragging "someday" into the present.

There were personal reasons wrapped around the decision, but underneath all of that was a simple thought: I didn't want to leave this one on the table. I didn't want to be the guy who always said "I've always wanted to fly" and never actually tried. If I was going to stick around after almost dying, I wanted the time to mean something.

So I did what I always do when a big goal shows up. I started working the problem.

I did the research. I made calls. I talked to people who knew how the FAA really works. I asked what it would take, as a post-CABG heart patient, to get medical clearance for even a basic private pilot license. Not a fighter jet. Not an airline cockpit. Just a small plane, clear sky, left seat.

Because of my cardiac history, I didn't get to be the guy who just signs up for ground school and figures it out later. I had to jump through extra hoops before anyone would even consider me for a medical certificate. The big one was the stress test. I had to pass the Bruce Protocol on a treadmill: hit the required heart rate, hold it, and prove my patched-up circulatory system could handle the load.

So instead of buying a stack of pilot manuals right away, I went back to square one: my body.

I started training. Especially on the treadmill. Not glamorous, not Instagram content, just a guy in a gym trying to get his post-surgery legs and lungs to agree with each other. Before Christmas that first year, I couldn't even do a decent modified push-up. My chest was still temperamental, my arms were weak, and my sternum had Opinions about sudden movement. Now I was aiming at a test designed for healthy people, not guys who'd had their chest opened.

Eventually, it was time for the real thing.

This wasn't the casual treadmill in the corner

of the cardiologist's office. This was the full setup: EKG, nurse, tech, wires everywhere. Stickers on my chest. Blood pressure cuff. Baseline readings. I lay on my left side while they took pictures of my heart from different angles to get a clean "before" view.

I warned them going in: my blood pressure runs hot. It always has. The surgery fixed the plumbing, but my system still likes to run in the high-normal range even on a good day. Now, at least, the blood moving through the pipes was fully oxygenated instead of squeezing through compromised blockages. Clean fuel in, stronger pump.

The Bruce Protocol ramps in stages. Every few minutes, the treadmill speed and incline go up. You either keep up or tap out.

My run lasted about twelve minutes.

I did what I do when I'm under stress: I talked.

I kept up a running commentary with the nurse and the tech. Part of that was just me being me—I crack jokes when I'm uncomfortable and I like making friends with medical staff. But part of it was intentional. If I could talk, read the inspirational posters on the wall out loud, and make snarky comments about them, that meant my brain was getting enough oxygen and my vision wasn't tunneling. I'd point to a sign and read it just to prove I was still fully online.

In the back of my head, another thought ran

quietly: if things go sideways—if my heart rhythm looks bad or my blood pressure spikes into the danger zone—they'll hit the stop button. They didn't. They just watched me sweat and climb the invisible hill.

By the time I hit the required workload, my left knee started complaining. Old injuries, old mileage. I looked at the nurse and basically said, "Okay. I passed. I'm done." There was no extra credit for blowing out a joint.

They moved me back to the table for the post-stress imaging. More pictures from different angles. This time, they weren't just watching motion; they were looking for ischemia—whether parts of my heart muscle were starving for blood under stress and whether they recovered afterward.

My rebuilt system did exactly what it was supposed to do. No ischemia. No hidden failure. Just a strong heart with better plumbing, pumping clean fuel the way it was designed to, and a guy who desperately needed a towel.

After that, I saw my new cardiologist. He went through the data, looked at me, and did the classic cardiologist two-step: "You did great. You passed. Also, you're still too heavy. Lose more weight." Then he smiled and said the part that mattered: "You did it, Robert."

Medically, the box was checked. I had passed the Bruce Protocol. I had the images and numbers to prove that my heart could handle stress. I had done the work.

From there, it was supposed to be straightforward. Submit the results. Gather the medical documentation. Let the FAA do their thing. Move on to the fun part: actually learning to fly.

Then the universe laughed.

Ascension—the health system that owns St. Mary's—got hammered by a cyberattack that took a wrecking ball to their electronic records. Systems went down. Hospitals went to paper workflows. Doctors and nurses were busy trying to keep the day-to-day medical chaos under control while IT teams scrambled behind the scenes.

I had my test done. I had my cardiologist's blessing. What I didn't have was a clean, functioning pipeline for getting those records from "inside a compromised hospital network" to "on an FAA medical examiner's desk in an acceptable format."

I requested records. I followed up. I made calls. I did the polite-pest thing everyone does when they're stuck inside a big system: "Just checking in on the status…" People were kind. People were stressed. People were working under conditions they didn't sign up for.

Meanwhile, the FAA clock kept ticking.

I applied for an extension. Got it. Waited some more. The records still didn't show up in the way the FAA needed them, in the timeframe I had.

My deadline passed.

And just like that, my shot at getting that pilot's medical—at least in that window—was gone. Not because I failed the test. Not because my heart couldn't handle it. Not because I blew off the requirements. Because a hospital network got punched in the mouth by a cyberattack and the paperwork pipeline collapsed.

Fuck my life.

This is the part people don't like to talk about, because it feels unfair and unfixable. Sometimes you do everything right and still lose. You train. You comply. You execute. You hit the numbers. And the result still comes back as "No" because of a variable you never touched.

That's not failure. That's just reality.

The outcome isn't always in your hands. You can engineer the hell out of your inputs, but the system you live in is bigger than you are. There are dependencies you don't control: hospital networks, federal agencies, servers, timing, other people's emergencies.

What is in your hands is how you respond when the answer comes back "No" for reasons that make you want to scream.

I could have let it defeat me. I could have said, "What's the point? I try and I try and something always breaks." And to be honest, there were moments I felt exactly like that. I sulked. I swore. I threw a private little pity party and replayed all the things that could have gone differently.

But I didn't stop.

In 2025, I decided to write a book.

I had all the first-time author nerves—Will it

suck? Will anyone read it? Does anyone care?—
but I did it anyway. I sat down, opened a blank
document, and started telling the stories that had
been piling up in my head and heart for years. I
found my voice again. I published *Dark Recipe*.

One door closed. I opened another.

That's all any of us can do. The universe will
throw obstacles at you that make no sense: cy-
berattacks, medical complications, job losses, bad
timing, personal betrayals, systems that glitch
right when you need them to behave. You
cannot engineer your way around all of it.

What you can control is whether you keep
going.

I have a sign on my wall that says, "Take the
risk or lose the chance." I believe that—mostly.
But I'd add something: take the calculated risk.
Not risk for the sake of drama. Not recklessness
dressed up as courage. A thoughtful bet on yourself, knowing that even if you lose the specific
thing you were aiming at, you'll still find another
way forward.

Fuck my life.

Keep going.

That's the only answer I've found that works.

TWELVE

The Physical Reality

Nobody prepares you for what your body feels like after they put it back together.

You know they're going to cut you open. You know they're going to wire your sternum shut. You understand it intellectually. But understanding and experiencing are two different things.

Here's the reality: it's going to suck. For a while.

Your chest is held together with wire. It isn't "fused" the way you imagine a broken bone fusing. At first it feels more like it's held—secured—while your body tries to do the actual healing. Every bump in the road on the way home shoots through you. You sit rigid in the passenger seat, terrified that if you shift wrong, your sternum won't heal straight.

And then there are the places you didn't expect to hurt.

They needed conduit to reroute blood

around blocked arteries. In my case, that meant my legs. One of the common "borrowed parts" in bypass surgery is the great saphenous vein from the leg. They can take what they need from one leg, but they may prep both legs depending on what they expect to need when they get in there. I went in for what ended up as a double bypass, but I woke up with both calves paying rent anyway.

And there's the "mammary" part that people describe in weird ways—me included.

For a long time I said, "They took a vein from my left breast," because that's how it lodged in my brain: chest, left side, something harvested. What I understand now is that what's commonly used is the left internal mammary artery—an artery that runs along the inside of your chest wall. It's not breast tissue, and it's not a vein. It's more like they repurpose a built-in line that was already there and route it to where it's needed.

My body became a parts warehouse.

The incisions on my calves—I don't think they were sutured well. I still have scars today. They've faded, but they're there.

And the nerves? Some of them never came back.

Three years later, there are still numb spots on my calves. It's better than it was, but it's probably permanent. Dead zones where the nerves were cut and never fully reconnected. It doesn't ruin my life, but it's a strange souvenir. A reminder that "recovery" doesn't always mean "back to factory settings."

My chest is mostly back to normal now. The feeling returned. But for a long time, the skin was numb. You touch your own body and feel nothing. It's unsettling—like your body belongs to someone else.

And the muscle mass? Gone.

You come out of surgery weak. The drugs, the bed rest, the trauma—it all takes a toll. You look in the mirror and see someone you don't recognize. Smaller. Softer. Fragile.

It takes time to come back. A long time. You don't just wake up one day and lift what you used to lift. You claw it back, inch by inch. You go to do something simple—lift a bag of groceries, open a heavy door—and the power just isn't there. The hydraulic pressure is gone.

So you keep trying. Eventually, the strength returns. Not like before—maybe never exactly like before—but enough. Enough to feel like yourself again.

And here's something nobody warns you about: sneezing and coughing.

You know that feeling when a sneeze is coming? That little tickle. The buildup. The inevitability.

After chest surgery, that feeling turns into panic.

Because sneezing and coughing are full-torso events. Every muscle contracts at once, and when your sternum is wired and healing, it can feel like your chest is going to blow apart.

They give you a heart pillow—a small cushion you're supposed to hug against your chest when you cough. You press it tight, brace yourself, and pray.

It still hurts like hell.

Coughing is worse because it stacks. One cough leads to another. You're clutching that pillow, eyes watering, trying to get through it without imagining the wires snapping.

It gets better. Eventually, a sneeze is just a sneeze again. But for those first weeks? You dread it. You feel that tickle and think, *Oh no. Here it comes.*

And laughing. God, laughing.

One of the best things in the world—something that connects you to people, something that makes life worth living—becomes a punishment.

Someone cracks a joke. You start to laugh. And then your chest reminds you you're still under construction.

You try to stop yourself. You hold it in. But that almost makes it worse. The suppressed laugh turns into a cough, and now you're clutching your heart pillow, stuck between pain and the absurdity of it.

And if you're the kind of person who thinks farts are funny—and let's be honest, most of us are—you're in trouble.

Someone rips one. Your brain registers it as hilarious. Your chest registers it as a threat.

You try not to laugh. You fail. Now you're in pain because of a fart.

But it's not just laughing at farts. It's having them.

Any pressure change in your torso becomes a project. You feel gas building up and you think, *Okay, easy. Controlled release.* Sometimes that works. Sometimes it doesn't. Your ribs get sore from bracing. Your chest aches from clenching. It's a circus.

Sneezing. Coughing. Laughing. Farting. All the normal bodily functions you never thought twice about become events. Obstacles. Things to survive.

There are moments in those first weeks where you question everything. Where the pain and the indignity and the frustration make you think, *Was it worth it?*

But you will be glad you did it.

On the other side of all that discomfort is a life you almost didn't get to live. The pain fades. The ribs heal. The fear of a sneeze fades into the background. Eventually you can laugh again without clutching a pillow like it's a life raft.

You just have to get through it first.

You have to work the problem.

Your body just went through hell. It's not going to bounce back because you want it to. You have to push it—carefully. Walk the halls. Do the breathing exercises. Get out of the chair even when it hurts. Prove to your body—and to yourself—that you're not done.

Some things will come back. Some things won't. The numb spots on my calves might be there forever. That's out of my control. I had to accept it or let it drive me crazy.

Acceptance isn't giving up. It's acknowledging reality so you can move forward.

Your sternum will heal. Your scars will fade. The numbness might improve or it might not. The muscle can come back if you work for it. Some days will be better than others.

It's going to suck. Then it's going to get better. Then some days it'll suck again.

That's the deal. You signed up for it the moment you got on the table. Now you have to live with it.

Keep working it.

THIRTEEN

The Recliner

When I came home on January 24th, I didn't walk into my house. I docked into it. I went from hospital bed to car seat to front door to one destination: the recliner in our living room. That chair wasn't furniture. It was life support with upholstery.

In theory, it was temporary. A few days. Maybe a week. Long enough for the worst of the pain to settle down so I could get in and out of bed without feeling like my sternum was going to unzip itself. In reality, I lived in that recliner for close to two months.

People don't tell you that part. They talk about the surgery, the statistics, the heroic surgeon, the moment you wake up with tubes. They don't tell you about the chair.

Command Central

That first afternoon, my world shrank to a three-foot radius. If it wasn't within arm's reach, it might as well have been on Mars, so the recliner became Command Central.

On my right: the television remote, my phone, a laptop, a water bottle, a nest of charging cables, a notebook and pen, and the plastic incentive spirometer they told me to use ten times an hour. On my left: meds, tissues, a little trash bag, and the heart pillow they sent home with me—the one you're supposed to hug when you cough or sneeze so your ribs don't feel like they're ejecting through your skin.

That pillow is a weird object. It looks like something you'd buy in a hospital gift shop: soft, printed, vaguely cheerful. In practice, it's body armor. Every time you feel a cough coming on, you grab it, clamp it tight to your chest, lean forward as much as the wires will allow, and hope the whole system holds. The first time you sneeze, you find religion whether you believe in anything or not.

The goal was simple: don't move more than necessary, don't lift anything heavier than a gallon of milk—actually, don't even lift the gallon of milk—and keep the sternum as still as possible while the bone does its slow, quiet work. That meant the recliner had to be set up like an engineer's workstation. Inputs, outputs, contingencies. You place everything you might need exactly where you can grab it without twisting.

I didn't pick the recliner because I love recliners. I picked it because a bed was a non-starter for a while. After a sternotomy, lying flat feels like somebody parked a truck on your chest and then asked you to sit up without using your arms. Rolling onto your side—my normal sleep position—was out of the question. The bone needs weeks of minimal movement to start knitting, and every twist feels like you're testing the welds. Sleeping in a regular bed isn't just uncomfortable; it's a bad idea.

There's also the part nobody warns you about: the empty side of the bed. If you're used to sleeping next to someone, suddenly putting them in the bed alone while you're exiled to another room does something strange to your head. They're still there. You're still married. But now they go to bed without you, and you stay in the recliner, listening to the house settle. You tell yourself it's temporary—and it is—but it still feels like a fault line running through your routine.

The recliner solved the mechanics. I could sleep half-upright, wedge pillows around my arms, and stand up without torquing my chest. It didn't solve the mental part. Knowing my wife was in the next room, in the bed we'd shared for years, while I camped in the living room in front of the TV, made the whole thing feel more real.

Surgery had already rearranged my body. Now it was rearranging where I slept.

And then you drop something.

When the Remote Wins

If you've never had your sternum wired shut, you don't fully appreciate how evil gravity can be. You drop your phone between the cushions, and on a normal day you just lean forward, fish around, and get on with your life. In the recliner era, a dropped remote is a full-scale incident.

There's this special moment of dread when you hear that plastic clack as the remote slips past the edge of the cushion and disappears into the crack. You freeze. Not because you're fragile and dainty, but because you know what retrieving it would cost.

If someone is home, you swallow your pride and ask for help.

"Hey, can you grab that? It fell."

If no one is home, and you're still in the early weeks where every move feels like it tugs on the wires, you just lost entertainment, communication, or both. You're stuck staring at whatever channel you were on until somebody comes back, and hope to God it wasn't a home-shopping marathon.

Can you get out of the chair and get it yourself? Maybe. Depends on the day. Depends on the pain. Depends on how confident you are that your chest will tolerate the twisting and pushing required to stand up, dig around, and sit back down without something popping or tearing. Early on, the answer is no. Later, the answer is maybe, but you'll think about it longer than you ever thought about bending over in your life.

Little things like that start to mess with your head. You go from being a guy who runs companies and solves complex problems to a guy who is temporarily defeated by a La-Z-Boy and a television remote. It's humbling in the way a pie in the face is humbling. Not dramatic. Just absurd.

Temperature Wars

This was late January in Michigan. Our house isn't drafty by 1920s farmhouse standards, but it isn't a lab-sealed space capsule either. The recliner sat near a fireplace with a downdraft issue. On windy days, you could feel the air move in ways that didn't match the thermostat. The result was a constant low-grade battle for comfort.

Some days, my legs would be too warm. I'd kick the blanket off and instantly regret it. The air would hit my calves, travel up those angry incision lines, and my whole body would decide we were too cold. Then the blanket came back up. Ten minutes later, I was sweating again.

Your system is doing its own thing that first month. Your body is burning energy to heal bone and soft tissue, adjusting to new blood flow patterns, and processing whatever cocktail of meds you're on. Temperature control becomes another variable you can't quite dial in, and even adjusting blankets and socks turns into a project because you're too sore to move efficiently.

The drafts weren't life-threatening. They were just one more reminder that nothing was quite right. Not catastrophic, not unbearable— just off. All day. Every day.

The Bathroom as Field Trip

When your universe shrinks to a recliner, normal tasks take on a strange kind of glamour. Going to the bathroom becomes a highlight. Not because anything exciting happens in there, but because it's movement. It's a change in scenery.

Getting out of the chair is a whole procedure. You don't just pop up. You plan it. You plant your feet, scoot to the edge, keep your elbows tucked in so you don't torque your chest, and push with your legs, not your arms. Sternal precautions are clear: no using your arms to push yourself up, no heavy lifting, no flaring your elbows like you're doing a bench press with your own bodyweight.

By the time you're standing, you're already tired. You shuffle down the hallway at a pace that would annoy a turtle, do your business, wash your hands, and reverse the process to sit back down. Total distance traveled: maybe forty feet. Emotional impact: oddly huge.

I started to understand why older people

make such a big deal out of "taking a walk to the mailbox." When your body is limited, even small movement is an event.

My Wife the Nurse and Caretaker

Those first days home, my wife was still in full trauma-nurse mode, even though we were out of the hospital. She took my vitals. Checked my blood pressure. Watched my legs for pitting edema—pressing her fingers into my calves to see if the imprint stayed, a sign that fluid was building up where it shouldn't. She kept notes.

On January 31st, we took that little logbook to my first post-op appointment with the surgeon, twelve days out from the bypass. He flipped through the numbers, looked at the incisions, listened to my lungs, and nodded. On paper, the system was behaving.

I, on the other hand, was losing my mind.

The recliner had gone from lifesaver to prison cell in about seven days. I'm not wired to sit still. I have nervous energy under the best of circumstances. Now I was stuck in one spot, in one position, with a chest that couldn't be bumped, lifted, twisted, or trusted. It showed.

I told the surgeon I was going stir-crazy. Not bravely. Not dramatically. Just honestly.

He glanced at my chart, glanced at my wife's notes, and made a call that wasn't written on any form. He cleared me for limited driving. Not cross-country road trips. Not rush-hour highway battles. Just a couple miles to my office, straight shot, no heroics.

From a liability standpoint, that's a gray area. From a human standpoint, it was oxygen. Most guidelines say four to six weeks before driving after a median sternotomy, once the bone has had time to knit and reaction time is back. He looked at me, looked at the distance involved, and decided I was safe enough and sane enough to handle it.

That little bit of autonomy—being able to leave the house under my own power, even for a short drive—changed everything. I still spent most of my hours in that recliner, but now it wasn't the entire universe. It was home base.

Faster Than Expected, Slower Than I Wanted

Physiologically, I was ahead of schedule. My heart itself—the pump—was strong. The plumbing had been the problem. Once the blockages were bypassed and the grafts were in place, my circulation numbers improved faster than anyone expected for a guy my size.

One of our daughters came home not long after surgery. She'd been around hospitals too and knew what post-op cardiac patients usually look like. I think she was braced to see a gray, fragile, hollow-eyed version of her dad—

tube-ridden, withdrawn, maybe barely able to stand.

What she walked into instead was a man in a recliner who was annoyed more than anything. Sore, wired together, limited—but alert, talking, cracking jokes, complaining about the chair and the boredom. Not the ghost she expected.

That reaction told me something I couldn't see from the inside: my body was doing better than my head was giving it credit for. I was pissed off about limits, but I wasn't actually circling the drain. The system was rebooting.

The flip side is that bone does not care about your attitude. The sternum still needed those six to eight weeks of relative stillness to reach decent strength, and up to three months to really heal. No amount of impatience could negotiate that timeline. I wasn't allowed to lift more than ten pounds. A gallon of milk was still out of scope.

I could want to do push-ups all day long. My chest had veto power.

Push-Ups and Gravity

Before surgery, push-ups were one of those things I could always do. Even when I was heavier than I should have been, even when my cardio sucked, I could drop to the floor and crank out a respectable number. It was a quiet point of pride.

After surgery, I couldn't do one. Not a good one. Not a bad one. Zero.

The first time I tried was months later, well past the initial healing window, cleared by the surgeon to increase activity. I got down on the floor, hands placed, toes planted, and lowered my body maybe two inches before my chest let me know we were done here. The wires held, but my confidence didn't.

It took time—slow, incremental work—before I could do a single push-up. When it finally happened, it wasn't an Instagram-worthy moment. No music swelled. No audience cheered. I just felt my body go all the way down, all the way up, and thought, Okay. We're getting somewhere.

That's how a lot of recovery works. You measure progress in units nobody else can see.

Scars and Sunlight

The surgical team did a nice job on my chest incision. It's not pretty, exactly—no one is going to mistake it for abstract art—but it's straight, clean, and settled into a line that mostly disappears unless the light hits it just right.

My calves are another story.

There's no mistaking where they harvested veins. Those incisions never quite looked like they belonged on the same body as the chest work. They healed, but not gracefully. Maybe they could have been sutured better. Maybe my skin just had opinions. Either way, the result is a set of irregular scars that still catch my eye when I'm in shorts.

For a while, I was more conscious of those than the chest. You don't think much about how your legs look in bright sunlight until the scar tissue starts reacting to UV. Fresh scars are notorious for darkening, thickening, and generally looking worse if you cook them in the sun too early.

So I adapted. I bought a swim shirt for the chest, partly for modesty, mostly for protection. If we were outside, I kept the scars covered as much as possible. Not out of vanity—though nobody is thrilled about looking like a Frankenstein project—but out of maintenance. If I'm going to carry these marks for the rest of my life, I'd rather not make them angrier than necessary.

Over time, I got used to them. They're part of the map now. Lines added later.

The Chair That Overstayed Its Welcome

The strange thing is how fast you can go from loving something to resenting it.

In the early days, that recliner was my best friend. It was the only place I could sit, sleep, and shift position without feeling like my chest was going to split. I was grateful for it. If we'd had to improvise with a flat couch or a regular chair, the whole experience would have been worse.

But after weeks of living in that same spot—eating there, dozing there, sweating there, shivering there, waking up in the middle of the night to adjust the blanket, clutch the heart pillow, and try not to cough—I started to hate it.

I hated the way the cushions compressed under the same weight in the same spot. I hated the sound the footrest made when it went up and down. I hated the little voids where the remote could vanish. I hated the way my world shrank to whatever I could see from that one angle.

By the time I graduated back to my own bed and regular chairs, the recliner had served its purpose. It had done its job. It kept me elevated when lying flat felt impossible, held me steady while my sternum knit, and gave me a place to be weak without collapsing.

And I almost never sit in it now.

It's still there, in the house. Other people use it. Guests. Family. Grandkids. To them, it's just a chair. To me, it's a museum exhibit.

In case of open-heart surgery, break glass.

The Quiet Part of Recovery

If you're reading this from your own version of that recliner—stuck, sore, surrounded by remotes and chargers and pillows—it might feel like nothing is happening. Like your life has stalled and you're just wasting time while everyone else moves on.

You're not.

You're doing the unglamorous, invisible part of survival. Your bone is rebuilding. Your grafts are settling in. Your body is reprogramming itself to run on new plumbing. Your mind is trying to figure out what the hell just happened.

It's going to be boring. It's going to be frustrating. You're going to drop things you can't pick up. You're going to get too hot, then too cold. You're going to feel stupid for getting excited about a trip to the bathroom. You're going to love that chair and then never want to see it again.

That's okay.

You don't have to transcend it. You don't have to turn the recliner stage into a motivational poster. You just have to get through it.

Work the problem. Keep what you need within reach. Ask for help when you drop the remote. Do your breathing. Take your meds. Walk when you can. Rest when you have to. Let the chair do its job until you're strong enough to walk past it.

Then go live the life you bought by sitting in it.

FOURTEEN

Get Out of Your Own Way

Here's something that still amazes me: my body saved itself before anyone else could.

When my LAD was 99% blocked—when the main highway feeding my heart was almost closed—my body didn't just give up. It didn't throw an error message and shut down. It built a workaround.

Without me knowing, without me doing a damn thing, my body grew collateral circulation —extra pathways that let blood detour around a restriction. Not a perfect fix. Not a permanent solution. More like side streets and back roads that keep traffic moving when the interstate is a parking lot. It bought me time.

The surgeon showed me the images. He pointed at the screen with something close to reverence. "The body is a beautiful machine, Mr. Cummer. It grew these pathways to save you."

I didn't tell it to do that. I didn't even know it

was happening. My body just worked the problem in the background while I was busy ignoring the check engine light.

And to be clear: this wasn't magic. It didn't happen overnight. Those pathways develop over time in response to a problem—your body sensing starvation and adapting the only way it can. The point is still the same: while I was negotiating with reality, my body was already trying to keep me alive.

That's what the body does. And, in its own way, that's what the mind can do too—if you let it.

After surgery, your job is to get out of your own way.

That doesn't mean being passive. It doesn't mean lying in bed and waiting for healing to happen. You still have to do the work—the walking, the breathing exercises, the slow grind of strength returning. That part is on you.

But there's another part that isn't on you. The part where your body knits itself back together. The part where tissues heal, grafts settle in, swelling calms down, and your system adapts to the new routing. The part that happens on a schedule you don't control.

You have to let that happen.

I'm an engineer. I like to control variables. I like to understand systems and predict outcomes. Before all of this, if something was broken, the default wiring in my head said: find the root cause, change the inputs, fix the outputs. After surgery, I had to accept that some of the most important work was happening without my input.

My sternum was healing. My body was adjusting to new blood flow patterns. My nerves were trying to reconnect—some successfully, some not. All of that was happening in the background, on its own timeline, regardless of how badly I wanted to speed it up.

There's a strange kind of humility in realizing you can't "optimize" bone healing. You can support it. You can avoid doing dumb things. But you can't will calcium to deposit faster. You can't negotiate with scar tissue. You can't sprint through six weeks of recovery in three.

The same is true for your mind.

You just faced your own mortality. You lay on a table and let strangers stop your heart. That's not nothing. Your brain has to process that. It has to file it away, make sense of it, integrate it into who you are now.

That takes time. And it doesn't happen on command.

Some days you'll feel fine. You'll make coffee, answer emails, shuffle around the house, and think, I'm okay. I've got this. Other days, the weight of it will hit you out of nowhere. You'll be doing something mundane—washing dishes, driving to the store, folding laundry—and suddenly you'll think, Holy shit. I almost died.

Sometimes it shows up as what the professionals politely call "cardiac blues"—that weird mix of mood swings, brain fog, irritability, and sadness that comes after a big cardiac event. Not full-blown depression, just an emotional hangover from what your body and brain have been through.

Let it come.

Don't fight it. Don't tell yourself you "should be over it by now." That's you getting in your own way again. Your mind is working the problem, just like your body did when it built those detours around a failing artery. In plain English, your brain is rewiring itself around a trauma.

Here's where "get out of your own way" gets practical.

There are things you can control:

- You can show up for cardiac rehab or your version of it—walks, light exercise, following the plan—even when you don't feel like it.
- You can take the meds, even when you'd rather pretend you don't need them.
- You can keep your follow-up appointments and ask the questions that are bugging you.
- You can tell at least one person the truth when they ask how you're doing.

And there are things you can't control:

- How fast your sternum knits.
- How quickly your energy returns.
- How long it takes before a flight of stairs doesn't feel like a summit attempt.
- How long it takes your brain to stop replaying images of the OR and the "what if" scenarios at three in the morning.

If you try to white-knuckle the second list, you just increase your suffering. You start judging your healing like a performance review: Am I ahead of schedule? Am I behind? Am I doing this right?

Instead, try thinking about it the way your surgeon thought about those collateral vessels: as a system that's quietly, constantly working on your behalf, even when you're not paying attention.

Your job is to cooperate with that system, not fight it.

Work the problem where you can. Do the rehab. Take the walks. Breathe into the spirometer. Get stronger.

For the rest of it—the healing you can't control, the processing you can't force—get out of your own way.

Your body knew how to save you before. It

grew side streets and back roads around a traffic jam you didn't even know was forming. It kept you alive long enough for someone with a scalpel and a plan to get in there and fix the main route.

Trust it to finish the job now.

FIFTEEN

Finding Your It

There's a song called "Live Like You Were Dying." You've probably heard it. Tim McGraw delivered a beautiful anthem about a man who gets a terminal diagnosis and finally understands what matters—loving deeper, speaking sweeter, forgiveness.

It's a powerful song. It's about appreciation and reflection, and I respect the sentiment deeply.

But I have my own way of channeling that energy.

Sometimes, people hear that title and think it means they have to go chase adrenaline—skydiving, Rocky Mountain climbing, taking wild risks just to feel alive. They make a bucket list and start treating life like a stunt reel. I don't think the song is reckless, but I think the reaction to it can be if you aren't careful.

I'm not against adventure. I like a good thrill as much as the next person. But for me, there's a difference between taking a risk just to prove you're alive, and taking a calculated risk to build a life that's actually yours.

I have a sign on my wall: "Take the risk or lose the chance."

I believe that. But I'd add something: don't take the risk until you know what you're taking it for.

That's your "It."

Your It is the thing that makes your life feel like it's actually yours. The thing you'd regret not doing. The thing that matters even if nobody claps. The thing that pulls you forward when fear, inertia, or comfort are telling you to stay put.

For a long time, I expressed mine with my hands.

I've always enjoyed making things. Over the years, I remodeled every inch of my basement. I added a full bath with a custom tile enclosure. I built a full bar out of oak—sanding it down with 400-grit sandpaper because I was convinced that if I worked it hard enough, you wouldn't even be able to feel the seams.

I spent weekends at the table saw and evenings covered in sawdust. I'd obsess over tiny details that no casual visitor would ever notice: the way two boards met at a corner, the alignment of grout lines, whether the sheen on the bar top was perfectly even. That was my It at the time—taking raw materials and turning them into something real, something solid, something people could touch.

I'm an engineer, so perfectionism is just part of the specs.

But in 2025, I felt a shift. My It wasn't about wood or tile anymore. It was about writing.

It started quietly. A few notes. A few scenes. A sense that if I didn't get certain stories out of my head, they were going to sit there and rot. Writing became a way to express myself—to get the ideas and memories and what-ifs out of my internal hard drive and onto a page where I could actually do something with them.

It wasn't just creativity. It was maintenance.

Writing became essential. I had to write Dark Recipe. It wasn't a hobby; it was a compulsion. I can't even count the hours I poured into it. I'd work my normal duties as co-founder of Molly's Grape & Citrus Company, handle the operations, the logistics, the hundred little fires that pop up in a small business. Then I'd sit down at night, open the laptop, and write until two or three in the morning.

Here's the strange part: I was tired, but I wasn't exhausted.

There's a difference. Exhaustion is when your soul feels drained. This was just a body saying, "You're working hard," while the rest of me said, "Keep going." That's one of the signs you've found your It: the work costs you something, but you don't resent the bill.

Along the way, I started learning about the

publishing industry—specifically self-publishing. I learned what an "imprint" was. I learned how ISBNs work, how royalties get sliced up, how traditional contracts can take your rights and lease them back to you in tiny, controlled doses.

The more I learned, the more I realized I didn't want someone else's name on the spine of my work.

I didn't want to rent space in someone else's system. I wanted to build my own.

So I formed Mangrove Publishing Company. Right now, I'm its only writer, but I didn't create it as a vanity label. I created it as a home base—for my work, and eventually for the work of other people whose voices I believe in.

I chose that name for a specific reason.

As I looked at my life, I discovered that I had more than just blood family. I had a network of people who had held me up when things got dark. Friends, colleagues, extended family, people who showed up unasked. They weren't all connected to each other, but they were all connected to me. I kept picturing a mangrove forest—roots tangled together, stretching wide and deep, holding the shoreline in place when the tide tries to tear it apart.

Mangrove felt like the perfect name for a company built on that foundation.

Mangrove Publishing: where the roots run wide and deep. By blood, or by choice.

That, to me, is part of finding your It. It's

not just about what you do. It's about who you do it with, and who you do it for.

Your It doesn't have to be dramatic. It doesn't have to make a good story. It doesn't have to look impressive on social media. It just has to be true.

After surgery, you get a rare gift: clarity. For a little while, the noise drops and you can hear yourself again. You see what matters and what doesn't. You see who matters and who doesn't. All the bullshit filters fall away, and you're left with a handful of things that actually move the needle for you.

Use that clarity. Don't waste it.

Ask yourself: what do I want to go for? What have I been putting off? What would I regret not doing if time got cut short?

That's your It.

Maybe it's repairing a relationship. Maybe it's taking the trip you keep talking about. Maybe it's telling someone you love them without waiting for the "right moment." Maybe it's writing the book, starting the business, picking up the guitar again, learning to paint, changing a habit that's been quietly killing you.

Your It might be small from the outside. It might not look like much to anyone else. That's fine. This isn't a group project.

And your It can change over time.

The same guy who once found his joy in sanding oak bars now finds it in revising chapters and building a publishing imprint. Ten years from now, my It might shift again. That doesn't mean the old versions were wrong. It just means I'm still alive enough to evolve.

I'm not telling you to be reckless. I'm not telling you to empty your savings and jump out of a plane because a country song told you to seize the day.

I'm telling you to figure out what matters—really matters—and then go for it deliberately. With intention. With calculated risk.

Because "live like you were dying" isn't just about the dying part.

It's about living like you're living.

Find your It. Then, as much as you can, build your life around it.

SIXTEEN

Your Tribe

I chose the name Mangrove for a reason. Mangroves have roots that are wide and deep. They grow in harsh environments. They protect the shoreline. And they're interconnected—what looks like a forest of individual trees is actually a network, supporting each other beneath the surface.

That's how I think about family now. Not just blood. By blood or by choice.

Your tribe.

Over the years, my tribe has evolved. It had to. People come in and out of your life. Sometimes time just passes, or life gets busy, and you drift. It's natural. Jobs change. People move. Kids grow up. Health shifts. One year you're talking every week, and the next year you realize you've mostly been liking each other's posts instead of actually talking.

But I've also learned that "drift" doesn't mean "gone." The real ones are always part of your tribe, even from a distance. You might go months without a conversation, and then one text or one phone call snaps everything back into place like you saw each other yesterday.

I think I view connection differently because I experienced loss at an early age. When you lose people young, it wires you differently. You don't assume everyone will be there forever. You learn pretty quickly that the chair can go empty. You notice the spaces at the table where someone used to sit. You notice the phone that stops ringing.

Because of that, I tend to hold onto people a little tighter than expected. Maybe too tight sometimes. I'm the guy who checks in, the guy who worries, the guy who wants to make sure the circle is solid. I probably should let go a little more, but I don't like losing people. I know what that silence sounds like.

That instinct to gather people has shaped my whole life.

Some of my greatest memories aren't the perfect, Hallmark moments. They're the Thanksgivings where the table was crowded with non-traditional family members. Friends who didn't have a place to go. Neighbors who just fit in. People who were "part of us" even if they didn't share a last name.

I remember looking around those tables— the noise, the food, the mismatched chairs, kids weaving between adults, dogs lurking underfoot waiting for dropped turkey—and realizing that this was the point. I was part of them, and they were part of me. That meant something. It meant we weren't alone.

It wasn't about the perfect meal or the Instagram-ready table setting. It was about the fact that everyone in that room had chosen to be there. They could have stayed home. They could have said they were busy. Instead, they came, they contributed, they laughed, they listened. That's tribe.

Before surgery, I think I took that network for granted. Not intentionally. Just the way you do when you assume there's always more time. You figure you'll call them next week. You'll visit next month. You'll say the thing you need to say "when things calm down."

Then you're lying on a table with your chest cracked open, and "eventually" stops feeling guaranteed.

When I was in surgery, I didn't know who was in the waiting room. I was busy being unconscious. I found out later. It wasn't just the people I lived with. It was friends. Family. People I didn't expect. People who drove through a Michigan winter to sit in plastic chairs and wait to find out if I'd survive.

Nobody made them punch a time clock. There wasn't a sign-in sheet for "approved family only." They just showed up because that's what you do when someone in your tribe is on the table. You clear your schedule, you grab your keys, and you go sit under bad fluorescent lighting for however long it takes.

I'm not going to name them here. They know who they are.

That's your tribe. The ones who show up when it counts.

And it's not just the big moments—surgery days, funerals, crises. Tribe also looks like the friend who texts you on a random Tuesday because you crossed their mind. The neighbor who snow-blows your driveway while you're recovering. The coworker who quietly covers a meeting so you can make a doctor's appointment. The person who drops off soup on your porch and doesn't ring the bell because they know you're wiped out.

After surgery, I started noticing those gestures more. I also started noticing how often I'd told myself, "I need to reach out to so-and-so," and then didn't. That realization stung a little. I had spent a lot of time being grateful for my tribe in my head without always doing the work of being an active member of theirs.

So I made some changes.

I started telling people I loved them. Out loud. More often. Not just as a throwaway line at the end of a call, but in the middle of normal conversations. "Hey, I love you. I'm glad you're in my life." It felt awkward at first. Then it felt normal. Now it feels necessary.

I started checking in more. Not in a smothering way—I hope—but in a "You matter enough for me to make this call" way. A quick, "How are you, really?" A text that says, "Thought of you when I saw this," with a photo or a link attached. Small things, but intentional.

Because life is short, and I never want to wonder if I said the thing that needed to be said.

So I guess it was inevitable that I ended up here.

The company name—Mangrove Publishing —isn't just about publishing books. It's about creating with, for, and about my tribe.

When I picture Mangrove, I don't just see a logo or a stack of paperbacks. I see those Thanksgiving tables. I see waiting rooms. I see hospital hallways. I see living rooms full of people who chose to be there. I see roots under the waterline, tangled together in ways nobody on the surface can fully map.

Mangroves hold the shoreline in place when storms come. They keep the land from washing away. They create a safe harbor for all kinds of life that would otherwise be exposed and vulnerable.

That's what a tribe does.

Your tribe might look different from mine. You might have a big extended family, or a tiny one. You might have one or two close friends instead of a crowd. You might find your people in a church, a band, a book club, a gym, a group chat, a hobby you thought was just yours until somebody else lit up when you mentioned it.

It doesn't matter where you find them.

What matters is that you recognize who they are—and you treat them like the roots they are.

Check on them. Let them check on you. Invite them in. Accept invitations. Say the thing. Show up when it counts, and sometimes when it doesn't. Be honest. Be kind. Be willing to sit in the uncomfortable spaces, not just the celebrations.

This company, this name—Mangrove Publishing—is my way of planting a flag for that philosophy. It's a reminder, to myself as much as anyone, that none of us does this alone.

It's the roots that hold the whole system together.

SEVENTEEN

I Still Don't Know

I'm going to be honest with you: I don't have the answers.

I've written this whole book—shared my story, told you what I went through, offered what I learned—and I still don't know what the fuck is going on.

I don't know why my arteries clogged while other people smoke and drink and eat garbage and live to ninety. I don't know why my body grew collateral circulation that kept me alive long enough to get fixed, while Bruce's heart just wore out. I don't know why Craig died in his sleep a week before his fifty-fifth birthday.

I don't know if there's a God. I don't know what happens after we die. I don't know if Craig can see me writing about him right now.

I'm not against belief. I don't mock anyone who has faith. I just don't have certainty. And I'm not going to pretend I do.

What I do know is this: what I went through

changed me. Profoundly. I just can't fully explain it.

The appreciation I came out with—for life, for people, for moments—it's real. It's deep. But putting it into words is hard. It's not a slogan. It's not a bumper sticker. It's a shift in how I move through the world.

I notice small things more. Light on snow. The sound of my grandkids laughing in another room. The way my wife's voice changes when she goes from "on with the world" to "just us at home." The ordinary stuff that used to blur into the background now feels like evidence that I'm still here.

At the same time, some of the big things that used to get me spun up don't have the same grip anymore.

I still find politics fascinating. I've written novels that are political. I like talking about issues, examining how people think, understanding different perspectives. I can nerd out on policy all day if you let me. What changed is that I don't get flipped out about other people's views the way I used to.

I can disagree hard and still care about the person.

I've had friends for decades who are diametrically opposed to me politically. That's fine. We argue. We roll our eyes. We send each other articles to poke at the other side. But underneath all of that, the relationship matters more than the scoreboard. I've seen the scoreboard up close. It doesn't care about your talking points.

What I don't have patience for anymore is performance. Plastic people. People who recite sound bites instead of thinking. People who wear opinions like uniforms instead of arriving at them honestly.

Somewhere inside most people there are real views—authentic ones. Not the ones they post for likes. The ones they hold at three in the morning when they can't sleep. That's what I'm interested in. That's the kind of person I want to spend my time with.

Because time is finite. After you almost die, you stop treating your hours like they're an unlimited resource. You start paying attention. Who shows up. Who tells the truth. Who drains you. Who lifts you. Who actually listens when you speak and who just waits for their turn to talk.

You don't become perfect. You don't suddenly nail every relationship. But you do start making different choices.

You do your best. You adjust. You choose.

I was fortunate in one specific way: my pump was strong, even if the plumbing was a mess. That's why I bounced back. That's why Bruce didn't. Luck of the draw.

And that right there is the point: you don't get to control the hand you're dealt.

You can influence it at the margins—diet, exercise, stress, all the things cardiologists nag you about—but there's still a lot of randomness in the system. Genetics. Timing. What kind of help is available when you need it. Who's on shift that day. Whether someone recognizes what's happening fast enough.

The time you have left after surgery might be fifty years. It might be ten. It might be less. You don't get to know. Nobody does.

So use it wisely.

Spend it on people who matter. Pursue the things that mean something to you. Stop wasting energy on bullshit that doesn't move the needle. You don't have to live every day like a highlight reel. You just have to stop acting like you have infinite replays.

Here's something else I still don't know: I don't know if any of what I've written here will land the way I hope it does. I don't know if it will help you, or comfort you, or piss you off, or all three. I don't know if you'll see yourself in any of this.

But I know this is the truest version I can give you.

I still don't know what the fuck is going on. I don't have a neat philosophy or a tidy set of answers. I can't wrap this up in a bow and tell you that everything happens for a reason and here's the lesson.

What I can say is this: I know what's worth fighting for. I know who's worth my time. I know I almost didn't get this chance, and I'm not going to waste it.

That's enough for me.

Maybe it's enough for you too.

My father has a Rolodex of sayings. Two of them have stuck with me:

"Time waits for no one."

"The only thing certain in life is change. And that's subject to change."

He's right on both counts.

Nothing is guaranteed. Not your health, not your plans, not the people around you. The ground shifts. The rules change. What you thought was solid turns out to be temporary. And while you're figuring it out, the clock keeps ticking.

You don't get to hit pause just because you're confused. You don't get extra time just because you finally figured out what you should have been doing all along. The meter keeps running whether you're ready or not.

But that's not a reason to give up. That's a reason to keep moving.

Change is coming whether you're ready or not. Time is passing whether you use it or not.

The question is what you do with whatever you've got left.

You don't need certainty to answer that question. You don't need a full theology or a master plan. You just need enough honesty to say, "This is who I am. These are my people. This is what matters to me. This is what I'm going to do with today."

Make it count.

Whatever "count" looks like for you—love, work, service, creation, presence—lean into it. You're not going to solve the mystery of life in one sitting. Neither am I.

But we can both decide not to waste the part we've been given.

EIGHTEEN

Perspective Isn't a Contest

There are days I still feel sorry for myself.

I don't say that proudly. I say it because it's true. Some days the weight shows up anyway—fatigue, frustration, loneliness, the "why me" loop. The kind of day where your brain starts building a case against reality. You replay the medical charts, the "what ifs," the things you wish you'd done sooner. You look at the scars and think, I didn't ask for this.

And then I'll pick up a book like *Indianapolis* —the story of the USS Indianapolis disaster— and something in me resets.

You read about men left in the water for days. Wounded. Exhausted. Burning oil on the surface. Darkness at night. Sun during the day. No control. No rescue in sight. Some of them barely had time in the Navy before they were thrown into a nightmare they never signed up for. No choice, no preparation, no second opinion. Just impact, chaos, and survival.

And you can't help thinking, Jesus Christ… what am I feeling sorry for myself about?

That thought can sound harsh, even cruel, if you say it wrong. So let me say what I mean—and what I don't mean.

I don't mean your pain is fake because somebody else had it worse.

Your worst day is still your worst day.

Your fear before surgery was real.

Your recovery is real.

Your exhaustion, your anger, the days you don't feel strong—real.

Life is complicated. Trauma doesn't care about scoreboards. Your nervous system doesn't pull up a chart of human suffering before it decides whether to be overwhelmed. It just responds to what you've lived.

But perspective is still useful. Sometimes it's the only thing that snaps you out of self-pity long enough to stand back up.

Here's what that Indianapolis story does for me: it reminds me that life isn't fair, and it never promised to be. Bad things happen to good people. Randomness exists. Innocent people get crushed by circumstances they didn't choose. The world is not a neat system with clean inputs and predictable outputs.

It just is.

And as bleak as that sounds, there's a strange kind of freedom in it.

Because if the universe isn't fair, then I don't have to keep arguing with it like fairness is a con-

tract I can enforce. I don't have to keep replaying the same mental courtroom drama—I
did the right things, so I deserved a different outcome. I can drop that argument and put my energy where it actually matters.

What do I do now?

When I read about suffering on that scale, it
doesn't erase my problems. It doesn't magically
make grief disappear. But it does slap my perspective back into alignment. It reminds me that
I still have choices. I still have options. I still have
agency.

I wasn't left at sea.

I wasn't helpless.

I got to be treated. I got to go home. I got
another chance.

And if I'm honest, sometimes I need a blunt
reminder like that. Not because I'm weak, but
because humans drift. We spiral. We turn one
hard season into a permanent identity. "Heart
patient." "Widow." "Laid-off guy." "Divorced."
We start to believe that's all we are.

Perspective interrupts the spiral.

It doesn't have to come from tragedy, either.
It can come from watching someone else fight.
From hearing a friend's story about chemo.
From seeing what your parents survived when
they were young. From remembering what your
grandparents went through and never talked
about. From realizing your kids and grandkids
are watching how you handle pressure. From
catching yourself laughing on a day you thought

would be nothing but tears and realizing, Okay, maybe I'm not done yet.

Perspective isn't about minimizing your pain. It's about right-sizing it.

If you're reading this and you're in a rough stretch—pre-surgery, post-surgery, or just life doing what life does—here's the point:

Don't compare pain like it's a competition.

But do use perspective as a tool.

There's a difference between "Other people have it worse, so shut up," and "Other people have survived hell, so maybe I can survive this."

The first one is cruelty.

The second one is strength.

The first voice shames you for struggling. The second voice stands next to you and says, "Look. We're not the first ones to be knocked down. We won't be the last. But people have gotten back up from worse. Let's see what we can do with this."

That book about the Indianapolis reminds me that suffering isn't moral. It isn't assigned fairly. It isn't always earned. Sometimes you're just on the wrong ship on the wrong night. Sometimes you just drew the short genetic straw. Sometimes you did everything "right" and still got the bad news.

Which means the only sane move is to stop waiting for fairness and start building resilience.

Resilience doesn't mean pretending everything is fine. It doesn't mean smiling through pain or refusing to acknowledge how hard it is. It means you feel the hit, you acknowledge it, and you keep looking for the next step anyway.

Some days the most heroic thing you can do is not a dramatic transformation.

It's just this:

Get your shit together.

Take a breath.

Eat something.

Take the meds.

Make the phone call.

Walk to the end of the driveway.

Do the next right thing.

And keep going.

You don't have to win the suffering Olympics. You don't have to justify your pain by ranking it against someone else's. You just have to refuse to let it be the only story you tell yourself about your life.

NINETEEN

Built to Survive

Sometimes perspective doesn't come from comparing yourself to strangers.

Sometimes it comes from your own bloodline.

I've spent a lot of time studying wartime history—battles, campaigns, the kinds of events that leave permanent fingerprints on the people who lived through them. Part of that is just who I am. I'm an amateur historian. I'm wired to analyze. I want to understand how humans behave under pressure.

But part of it is closer than history books.

My paternal grandfather, Russell E. Cummer, was a World War II Marine and part of the first occupation of Guadalcanal. He survived that and came home and married my grandmother. My maternal grandfather, Robert Henderson, was a Marine too. Both of my grandfathers served in the Pacific theater. One way or another, they lived through things most of us can't truly imagine without turning it into a movie in our heads.

And then there's my father, Russell Edward Cummer II—combat in Vietnam in 196–1967, 1st of the 8th Air Cavalry. Jumping out of helicopters. Horrific battles. Seeing things you don't unsee.

I grew up with those facts in the background. Not as a constant lecture, not as a "you don't know how easy you have it" speech on repeat, but as part of the family wiring. Names, units, locations. A sense that the men who raised me had walked through fire, even if they didn't give me a blow-by-blow.

I think about them sometimes when I'm tempted to feel sorry for myself.

Not because I think my struggle is fake. Not because I think heart surgery is "no big deal." It is a big deal. It's terrifying. It's surreal. It changes you. You don't go under anesthesia while someone stops your heart and come back exactly the same person.

But remembering them reminds me of something simple: fear is universal. The situation changes, but fear is fear. It doesn't care if you're in a jungle, on a ship, in a hospital gown, or sitting in your living room waiting for a phone call.

And what matters isn't whether you were scared—it's what you did next.

I don't look at their experiences and think, I'm less of a man.

If anything, I look at their experiences and think: they were human beings doing human things under impossible pressure. They found a way to function. They found a way to keep going. And then they carried whatever they had to carry afterward.

Some people made it through war and never truly came home inside their own heads.

Some didn't make it through at all.

So when I say "we're built to survive," I don't mean it like a motivational poster. I'm not saying grit your teeth and hustle. I mean it like biology.

My own body proved it to me.

When my LAD was 99% blocked, my body didn't consult my opinion. It didn't wait for me to behave better. It didn't care about my denial. It adapted. It grew collateral circulation—workarounds—because somewhere deep in the system, the mission was still the same: survive.

My brain didn't sit there and consciously type code into my arteries.

But the system responded anyway.

That's what living things do.

Zoom out, and you see the same pattern everywhere. Not just in arteries, but in people.

My grandfathers. My father. People in wartime. People in hospitals. People in divorce. People in addiction. People in grief. People in the quiet battles nobody sees—the caregiver who doesn't sleep through the night for months, the single parent juggling three jobs, the person going to work every day with a loss no one at the office knows about.

The details are different, but the pattern is familiar: a human being under stress finding a way to keep moving.

Sometimes "built to survive" looks like a Marine on a Pacific island. Sometimes it looks like a guy shuffling around his living room with a heart pillow pressed to his chest. Sometimes it looks like simply getting out of bed on a day you don't want to be conscious.

Some days I feel like I owe it to them—my grandfathers, my father, the people who came before me—to put one foot in front of the other.

Not because they would shame me if I didn't.

Because they didn't get to quit either.

They carried weight I'll never fully understand, and they still got up the next morning and did what needed to be done. They raised families. They went to work. They showed up at birthdays and ballgames. They mowed lawns and fixed cars and sat at kitchen tables pretending everything was normal while parts of them were still in another country.

That kind of endurance echoes forward. It becomes part of your wiring—whether you call it family, resilience, faith, stubbornness, or just survival instinct.

I'm not claiming hero status. I'm not comparing a bypass to combat. I'm not doing that.

What I'm saying is this: adversity is part of

the human contract, and nobody gets the same version of it. Some people get physiology that buys them time. Some don't. Some people get support systems. Some don't. Some people get lucky. Some don't.

You don't get to pick which storm hits you. You only get to decide what you do once you're in it.

So when you're still here—when you've been given more time—you have a responsibility to use it.

To keep going.

To be present.

To love your people.

To do the thing you keep putting off.

To tell the truth.

To build something that matters, even if it only matters to one person.

Sometimes that "something" is a company. Sometimes it's a book. Sometimes it's a conversation you've been avoiding. Sometimes it's just making sure your grandkids know your stories while you're still around to tell them.

That's why I wrote this the way I wrote it—through my own lens, from my own memory, without pretending I have airtight explanations for everything.

Because we all see life through our own lens.

Your storms won't look exactly like mine. Your scars won't match mine. Your family history, your wiring, your circumstances—they're yours. But if anything in these pages helps you see your own capacity to endure, to adapt, to survive, then the lens did its job.

If what I've described here helps even one person take the next step—one foot in front of the other—then it was worth putting it on paper.

About the Author

Robert Cummer is an engineer turned novelist with more than three decades in industrial automation, process control, and large-scale engineered systems. His career spans engineering innovation, systems integration, cross-disciplinary R&D, and executive leadership in global operations.

Drawing on a lifelong love of history, espionage fiction, and big-stakes human stories, Cummer writes thrillers where technology shapes the world but never overshadows the people caught inside it. His novels blend layered systems, geopolitical pressure, and the messy perseverance of ordinary individuals confronting extraordinary circumstances. For him, technology isn't the story—it's the force that drives the story forward.

Cummer is co-founder and CTO/COO of Molly's Grape & Citrus Company, where he oversees technology, digital infrastructure, and food-safety programs. A Michigan native, he holds multiple U.S. patents and has spent his career solving complex engineering challenges.

He is also the founder of Mangrove Publishing, an imprint dedicated to stories where the roots run deep.

Also by Robert Cummer

<u>Knox Ramsey Thrillers</u>

Dark Recipe

Terms & Conditions

(Coming Summer 2026)

<u>Boots on the Ground Series</u>

Instrumentation & Sensors: Field Guide

(Coming Spring 2026)